THE GOOD ENOUGH DIET

Where near enough is good enough to lose weight

TARA DIVERSI & DR ADAM FRASER

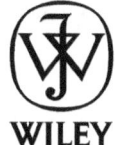

WILEY

John Wiley & Sons Australia, Ltd

First published 2011 by John Wiley & Sons Australia, Ltd
42 McDougall Street, Milton Qld 4064

Office also in Melbourne

Typeset in ITC Giovanni 10.5/13pt

© Tara Diversi and Adam Fraser 2011

The moral rights of the authors have been asserted

National Library of Australia Cataloguing-in-Publication data:

Author:	Fraser, Adam.
Title:	The good enough diet: where near enough is good enough to lose weight / Adam Fraser, Tara Diversi.
ISBN:	9780730375722 (pbk.)
Notes:	Includes index.
Subjects:	Weight loss.
	Reducing diets.
Other Authors/Contributors:	Diversi, Tara.
Dewey Number:	613.25

All rights reserved. Except as permitted under the *Australian Copyright Act 1968* (for example, a fair dealing for the purposes of study, research, criticism or review), no part of this book may be reproduced, stored in a retrieval system, communicated or transmitted in any form or by any means without prior written permission. All enquiries should be made to the publisher at the address above.

Cover design by Studio131 <www.studio131.net>

Cover image © istockphoto.com/Misko Kordic

10 9 8 7 6 5 4 3 2 1

Disclaimer

The material in this publication is of the nature of general comment only, and does not represent professional advice. It is not intended to provide specific guidance for particular circumstances and it should not be relied on as the basis for any decision to take action or not take action on any matter which it covers. Readers should obtain professional advice where appropriate, before making any such decision. To the maximum extent permitted by law, the authors and publisher disclaim all responsibility and liability to any person, arising directly or indirectly from any person taking or not taking action based upon the information in this publication.

Dedication

For Mike and Diane, who have always enthusiastically supported me in following my dreams ~ T.D.

For Dougie and Di, who are the perfect embodiment of love, support and devotion ~ A.F.

Contents

About the authors   vii
Acknowledgements   ix
Introduction: Is near enough good enough to lose weight?   xi

1 New world, new rules   1

Part I: Good enough diet

2 Proactive eating   7
3 The main ingredient   15
4 Variety   23
5 Comfort food   31
6 Is low-fat food making you fat?   39
7 Think before you drink   47

Part II: Good enough exercise

8 Productive exercise   57
9 Your exercise profile   65

10	The best exercise	75
11	Anytime is the right time	87
12	Have fun with it	97
13	Dress for success	105

Part III: Good enough mindset

14	Positive mindset	115
15	It's okay to be fat	123
16	Exercise and the third space	129
17	It's okay to be hungry	135

Part IV: Good enough mythbusting

18	Demystifying myths	145
19	Food combining	151
20	Feel free to have three	157
21	A fast game's a good game	163

Part V: Good enough in real life

22	Health in a hurry	171
23	Travelling success	185
24	Fit families	199

Endnote	207
Appendix A: Non-starchy vegetables and fruits and free flavourings	209
Appendix B: Drinks and their kilojoule content	211
Appendix C: Example meal plans	217
Appendix D: The hotel room workout	225
Appendix E: Metric to imperial conversion chart	229
Index	231

About the authors

Tara Diversi is an accredited practising dietitian with additional training in psychology and business. She has helped over 6000 clients on their weight loss journeys. As well as her Masters of Nutrition and Dietetics, Tara holds a Graduate Diploma of Psychology and an MBA. She is a lecturer at the University of Sydney and her business, Health Management Dietetics, is located in Cairns. She regularly provides expert comment for the media and is a spokesperson for the Dietitians Association of Australia.

Dr Adam Fraser is an accredited exercise physiologist with a PhD in Metabolism and Glucose control. He is the CEO of The Glucose Club, a company that guides and supports individuals towards a lifestyle that will improve their quality of life and their mental and physical wellbeing. Each day The Glucose Club works with some of Australia's most influential business leaders to keep them at the top of their game. Adam is the author of the best-selling book *Sugar Daddy*, which focuses on the lifestyle management of diabetes. He is also one of Australia's most in-demand presenters. In the last five years he has delivered more than 600 presentations to over 50 000 people. Most importantly he is married to a woman who is far brighter than he is.

Acknowledgements

This book would not have been possible without the help and support of many people.

The support we receive from our families is amazing. We often argue about who has the most wonderful, supportive and generous parents. We agree that we are both very lucky to have Doug and Di Fraser and Mike and Diane Diversi on our sides, and they have always surrounded us with opportunities, sporting activities, education, kindness and, most importantly, love.

Christine Armarego made this book better. She has been a fantastic supportive wife to Adam and friend to Tara. She helped with research, writing and sharing ideas throughout the process. She is a brilliant exercise physiologist and her experience with clients was also very helpful.

We feel lucky to have had Mary Masters work with us to refine our ideas and develop them into a workable manuscript and book. Thank you to the team at Wiley, including Kate, Kristin, Georgie and Elizabeth, who all gave valuable suggestions and support throughout the publishing process.

Our title fits the personality and attitude we wanted for our book exactly. We have Matt Holt to thank for this, as well as for giving us invaluable advice throughout. Callan Taylor brought the book to life with a wonderful cover concept that conveys the sentiment of the book.

Thanks also to Julie Winterbottom from O2 Speakers for her enthusiasm, diplomacy and support, and to Kate Faber, Meghan Hall and Melissa Carmody: three incredible practitioners who helped with research and who will make a positive difference in the health world as their careers develop.

Friends who supported us through the journey include in particular Peter Sheahan, Shannon Meiklejohn, Campbell Pool, Neisha Graham and Meika Foster, who would listen to different parts of the book as it unfolded, as well as our trials and tribulations, and still act interested throughout the process.

We would also like to thank colleagues at the Human Nutrition Unit at the University of Sydney and Health Management Dietetics. In particular, we would like to mention Camey Demmitt and Kate Rogers, senior dietitians whose experience helped refine some of the concepts within this book.

Last but not least we would like to thank the clients who were a source of inspiration for this book, particularly those who allowed us to share their stories to help inspire others.

Introduction:
Is near enough good enough to lose weight?

You are busy.
You are working.
You are travelling.
You are looking after children.
You are completing extra study.
You are stressed.
You are enjoying life.
You are trying to be healthy.

Oh, there it is — *trying*...

You should lose weight.
You should eat better.
You should eat less takeaway.
You should eat less, period.
You should exercise more.
You should walk instead of driving.
You should get up early to exercise.
You should drink less alcohol.
You should drink more water.
You should sleep six to eight hours per night.

You are trying to lose weight but...

When you're busy there's no time.
When you're working you have social functions.
When you're travelling you eat conference food.
When you're with the kids they need treats.
When you're studying you can't exercise.
When you're stressed you emotionally eat.
When you're enjoying life you want to relax with your food and alcohol.
When you're trying to be healthy, trying to lose weight — you can never seem to be perfect all the time.

So, this is why you can't lose weight, right?

Wrong!

What's wrong with dieting today?

Dieting thrives on making us feel like failures. We switch on and off our diets with every little circuit break that comes along, like a work meeting or a birthday celebration.

We know that weight loss means you're either a success or a failure. But what if you could strive for something in between? Something that allowed you to still lose weight and still be healthy while achieving your career, financial and personal goals. What if you could really have your cake and eat it too!

There are over 30 000 copyrighted diets on the market, and although individual countries produce guidelines for healthy eating, they tend not to give a prescription for weight loss. So how do you know what is the right diet regimen for you? Is it the one you have tried before, where you *successfully* lost weight only to put it all back on again — with added interest? Is it the new diet that promises the world due to the new findings on how your body *really* works? Is it the one produced by someone who has been exactly where you have been and managed to lose weight? Or is it the one endorsed by a celebrity who has the body you aspire to create for yourself?

Unfortunately, if there were one *right* diet for everyone, there would be no need for us to write this book.

The traditional all or nothing approach

Matt Cooper is the type of guy we can all look up to. He has had a number of successful careers, and when switching careers from accounting to real estate, he used his combination of book smarts, street smarts and charisma to become one of the most successful real estate agents in Australia. He has received real estate awards within numerous companies, including worldwide accolades. In other areas of his life, Matt is also fortunate. He has a wonderful wife, Tammy, who works alongside him in their business. He has a strong group of friends, and has been able to enjoy travelling throughout the world.

One day Matt described his situation perfectly. 'My life is like Trivial Pursuit. I have the circular piece and all of my wedges are full. All of my wedges are flourishing... except one. My weight. I just can't seem to win that wedge, but when I do, it will be like I have all of my areas sorted.'

Matt is a smart, funny guy, but one thing for sure is that he's an all or nothing guy. He's tried just about *every* diet and weight loss program you could imagine. Initially, he would always lose weight. After a few months of his weight going down, something would happen. Don't get us wrong, there was some big stuff that would spike up in his life, and this was followed by falling off the wagon. Matt would slowly regain the weight he'd lost and go back to square one. He's fortunate enough to function at high levels — which we call percentages — in other areas of his life, and wanted his physical health and weight loss to be 100 per cent as well.

We would discuss this at length, and Matt would always want to do more, lose weight faster and be lighter than our expectations. This would ultimately lead to continual hiccups, frustrations and then weight gain. We knew Matt could lose weight. If only he would focus on being 60 per cent rather than 100 per cent. If only Matt would focus on being good enough.

> *The traditional all or nothing approach (cont'd)*
>
> Instead, to our frustration, Matt decided to take six months off work completely, exercising for as many hours as he could per day and eating as little as he could. He was training like an endurance athlete, and eating like a ballerina. Of course he was shedding the kilos. But what else in his life was he shedding? We would explain to Matt that life balance is easy when you concentrate on work *or* your diet, but the challenge is to get them to work together. But for Matt, as life went on, things would continue to get in the way of his 100 per cent ideal, and instead of stepping over the barrier, he would go back to his old ways.
>
> After six months of dieting and exercising, Matt was lighter and healthier, and his weight continued to drop. There were a few wild peaks when he did put on a lot of weight, but he was still 30 kilograms lighter than when he started. This frustrated Matt. He wanted to lose weight faster and he felt that his problem was not being perfect enough.
>
> Truth is, Matt is an all or nothing guy, swinging between 100 per cent perfect and 20 per cent perfect. When he got the balance, the balance that is achievable with the Good Enough Diet, Matt was able to lose weight without losing his life. It took a massive shift in his mindset, and there were hard times, but the longer we have kept at it, the weight has shifted and stays off. Matt is like many of our clients, who have everything sorted, but not their weight. We have written this book for people like Matt, so once and for all you can feel on top of every wedge in your life.

Do those who diet lose more weight?

If you have ever been in hospital, you know that registered nurses have a busy job. They enjoy the trials and tribulations of working in a caring profession and are stereotypically women, often with a family at home. Despite a relatively physical working environment where they are on their feet for an entire shift, they have similar levels of overweight and obesity as those outside the nursing profession. Dr Bruce Zitkus, a nurse practitioner and Professor at Stony Brook University, studied over 700 nurses to see whether their personality type affected their weight and weight loss efforts. Although there was no significant difference between the personality types, interestingly, Zitkus found that those who followed a diet regimen were significantly less likely to be successful in weight loss. How could this be?

How we will make weight loss achievable for you

Let's face it. We know you're not stupid. You know you're not stupid. You know the answer to weight loss. You don't need some diet expert or book to tell you what you are doing wrong. You know why you're not losing weight, don't you?

Within the diet and exercise sections of this book, we won't be telling you exactly what you should eat and what type of exercise you should be doing. Instead, we'll share with you the most important things you need to do to lose weight. There will be no last supper, there will be no starting next week, month or season. We've included strategies that you can implement straight away. You don't even need to have finished the whole book before you can begin. You can focus on one chapter at a time. We've included some sample menus and exercises, but these are just examples of what have worked for others. Feel free to use our examples, or choose something that meets our guidelines and integrates perfectly with your lifestyle.

Just because it's good for them, it might not be good for you

Do you ever wonder if dietitians, exercise physiologists, personal trainers or doctors follow the regimen they have prescribed for you? Do you ever feel jaded when you see the thin person indulging in the good things in life when you feel restrained?

What is most important is to decide where you want to be on the health and/or thinness scale. Truth is that if you're a photographic model, TV celebrity or Olympic athlete, your diet really does need to be nearly perfect to reach your life goals. When your job is to look perfect, you need to put the effort in to make your body perfect. That's what they are paid for. However, if you're an executive, businessperson or working in some kind of profession, chances are that your career success is not as highly weighted towards your body fat percentage.

Physical health, weight loss and their role in life balance

Physical health contributes to just one area of overall health and happiness. Some of our clients have put 100 per cent into their diet and fitness regimen, and despite achieving their physical health goals, end up suffering huge ramifications in other areas of their life such as career, relationships and social wellbeing. When people think of balance, or work–life balance, they tend to overly focus on physical health and spiritual health. This creates just as much of an inbalance as a person who solely focuses on improving their career. A strong overemphasis on physical health isn't a balanced approach, and may in fact be detrimental to your career, social health, financial health, spiritual health and/or community health—all of which are essential for our complete wellbeing.

You don't need to be a rocket scientist to know that the nutritional aspect of food is only one component of its role for us in the world. How often do you attend a social or work function or other celebration where food isn't involved? You can't hide away from this forever, and if you do, other areas of your health will suffer.

Losing weight without losing your life

If you want to lose weight, you need to decide on where you feel your physical health is at the moment, with 0 per cent being very unhealthy—characterised by no physical activity and little regard for nutrition in your meals — and 100 per cent characterised by completing over two hours of physical activity per day and eating *no* food that is classified as unhealthy.

As we discussed earlier, a 100 per cent ideal is required if your body is your currency, for example if you are an athlete or a model. For the rest of us, use the scale like scores at university. A pass conceded is at 40 per cent, a regular pass is 50 per cent, a credit is 65 per cent, a distinction is 75 per cent and a high distinction is 85 per cent.

Just like at university, if you want your score to increase, the time and energy you need to allocate to your healthy diet and exercise plan also needs to increase. But does dieting and exercising really have to be that regimented? Do we really have to exercise at a gym or start running kilometres every day just to shed some kilograms?

Perfectly healthy without being perfect

You can be perfectly healthy living at about 65 per cent, just like a credit average at university is perfectly respectable for further study or career advancement. You may only need to make some small changes to your diet and exercise to move up the ladder and lose weight. Many healthcare practitioners, including doctors, personal trainers and dietitians, weight loss programs or diet books will promote an idealistic '100 per cent' diet and exercise plan for you to lose weight. Because this lifestyle aligns well with their career and social goals, they may be living at this level themselves; however, if you were a fly on the wall, you would probably find that these professionals live at about 70 per cent to 80 per cent themselves. And that is perfectly okay.

The scale shown in table 1 is useful not only to track your physical health but for all areas of your life that contribute to your health as well. Where do you think you fall on this scale in terms of your current health and weight?

Table 1: where do you sit on the health and weight spectrum?

0%	10%	20%	30%	40%	50%	60%	70%	80%	90%	100%
Very unhealthy										Extremely healthy
Extreme weight gain										Extreme weight loss

Broad categories

We all have many aspects to our lives that are important to us. These can be broken into broad or specific categories. Figure 1 (overleaf) shows some broad categories that make up your life. By examining what is significant to you, you will be able to determine how much emphasis you can give to your diet and exercise regimen.

You can make broad categories — like the areas of health listed in figure 1 — or you can break them down into actual priorities and values that are important to you. For example, you could indicate nutrition and exercise separately. The nutritional aspect of your diet could be at 80 per cent, so you only need to exercise at 50 per cent. Other more specific priorities and values may be important to you, and it is always best to choose the three most important values in your life as well as the other broad areas that we have listed. Some examples you could include are: nutrition, exercise, sport, working hours, responsibility at work, work functions, organising extra activities at work, travel, eating out, going out at night, quiet catch-ups with friends, participating in hobbies, attending church, meditation, yoga, professional development, reading, formal courses, mentoring, romantic relationships, parental relationships, relationships with friends, volunteering, participating in events.

Figure 1: broad categories

Physical health	0% _____	100%
Career health	0% _____	100%
Social health	0% _____	100%
Spiritual health	0% _____	100%
Learning health	0% _____	100%
Relationship health	0% _____	100%
Community health	0% _____	100%

When you have defined your three most important specific areas and the other broad areas of your life, it is important to align them with your values. On a separate sheet of paper, list the categories and decide on a score that you would give yourself for each of these areas at the moment. Then decide on the score you would like to achieve.

Your balance bar graph

Now that you have defined your own broad categories, we call this your balance bar graph. The temptation is to make the percentages for all of the categories increase; however, there may be some areas that you need to pull back a little on so your balance bar graph aligns with your goals and values. It is also important to ask yourself how realistic your changes are, and never try to jump more than 30 per cent if your starting point is below 50 per cent, or more than 20 per cent if your starting point is above 50 per cent. This will happen naturally if you are an all or nothing type person, so be aware that you will be setting yourself up for failure.

Your balance bar graph is great to look back on, particularly when you are trying to decide what you should do at a certain point, or you find yourself giving too much in one area and not enough in another. You may be able to combine a couple of categories and get the benefits for two parts of your life in one activity, or you may find that you are self-sabotaging by unnecessarily concentrating on a category of lower importance.

To improve your attitude towards dieting and to get the best from this book, you will be able to look at your nutrition and exercise bar graphs and realise how far you need to go. If you are at 0 per cent now, you will be able to lose weight at 30 per cent. If you are currently at 60 per cent, you may need to go to 75 per cent or 80 per cent to lose weight.

This is the truth. You can lose weight without being perfect all the time. We can lose weight by doing small things. Losing weight can happen when your diet and exercise regimen is good enough, not perfect. Who would have thought that to lose weight, near enough may actually be good enough?

At different stages in your life, your balance bar graph will change. If you have a family, your priorities will be skewed towards parental relationships and responsibilities. Usually this focus will have an impact on other areas of your life, such as your career health, physical health and social health — this is okay. If you are just beginning your career, you may need to put additional focus on your career health and learning health. This focus may have a negative impact on other areas of your life, such as physical health, relationship health and community health — this, too, is okay.

The trouble begins when you become overly focused on one area because it was needed at a certain time and stage in your life. When life moves on and your situation changes, the habits created from this previous time may be hard to break, so reassessing every now and again is helpful, otherwise the world will let you know in a different way. For example, if you focus too much on parenting by giving up your own identity and needs long after your children need your undivided attention, then your physical health is bound to be affected. This is something we commonly see in our clinics — don't worry, the guilt will pass, and your children will be happier to have a healthy parent. We also see the busy career person who puts their work over everything. Amazingly they are surprised when they are diagnosed with type 2 diabetes or heart disease.

Great is the enemy of good!

When you work closely with people and their personal issues, such as their health, you find that they grow close to you and often open up about different aspects of their lives. Having worked one on one with thousands of people over the last 10 years we have lost count of how many have broken down in a session and divulged specific details about their lives that they may have never shared with anyone before. Their outburst is often followed by 'I'm sorry, I'm just a little bit stressed'. However, it's not stress that leads to these outbursts, rather an amazing amount of self-imposed pressure to be perfect in every aspect of their lives.

We see working mothers who think they *must* organise the household, pay all the bills on time, keep an immaculate home, raise perfect well-mannered children, keep their husbands satisfied, achieve great results at work, be charming, have loads of energy, look a million bucks, stay slim and never age.

We see men who are trying to cope with a world that has dramatically changed. They are expected to get in touch with their feelings, know how to relate to women, communicate with their wives about their problems, be an unselfish lover, understand the new generation, learn how to deal with new technology, pay for their kids' school fees, tackle the mortgage, implement brilliant strategies at work, cope with change in the workplace, be an inspiring leader, have a stomach like a six pack and look like Sean Connery when they reach 60.

This pressure is trickling down to our children. The US Department of Health and Human Services has shown that 80 per cent of girls in grades 3 to 6 are unhappy with their body shape. Many children are so busy they need personal organisers to ensure they attend all of their extracurricular activities. Four and five year olds spend more time in structured activities than they do in unstructured play. Why? Because of our desire to be perfect.

This desire to be great at everything is making us freakin' miserable!
Great is the enemy of good!
There are some parts of your life where you have to settle for good not great. Sometimes something has to give. Essentially this is the philosophy of our book — to lose weight you don't have to be perfect, you just have to be good enough. Insisting that your health is perfect will lead to worse results and a huge amount of unhappiness. This is one of those times where good enough is exactly that.

Throughout this book we are going to give you some tough love and realistic advice on what you need to do to lose weight. We will also help you to understand what really is good enough and what may simply be overkill when taking into account your individual lifestyle.

Chapter 1

NEW WORLD, NEW RULES

The world is getting faster and faster, and shows no signs of slowing down. For example, it's easy to forget how slow dial-up internet used to seem and now even broadband isn't fast enough for us. We even recently overheard someone in the lunchroom complaining about the fact that two-minute noodles actually take three minutes to make!

How our expectations have changed

Today our expectations are high. One thing particularly true is that we expect to get things instantaneously. With a click of a button and a few electronic forms completed, there is no reason to wait for anything today. It's a shame that our physiology hasn't changed as quickly as technology. If only weight loss were as easy as a flick of a switch. But this doesn't stop us, and many of our clients, searching for the quick fix. Even prescription weight loss pills and weight loss surgery require time and commitment.

Many of us consider technological advances as a source of dissatisfaction, barriers to getting anything done, and barriers to weight loss. Instead of using technologies available to us to help us lose weight, we waste time, mostly on the internet, looking for things that are relatively insignificant for losing weight — this bean, that spice or the magical fruit. Other times we look for products or medications that don't exist, but we still look. 'Surely there is a weight loss secret pill in some exotic country that no one has told me about yet.' You convince yourself as yet more time passes that you could have been doing something proactively for your weight.

Focus on a glass half full

We are too quick to judge the changing world as bad, and blame it for our weight gain, but there are some choices we can make when faced with this new world. For some people, going back to the old ways of dieting — weighing all your food, counting kilojoules, hitting the gym — and focusing on our physical health as a number one priority may work. For many others, it is the reason they fail.

The new world is here and, yes, it has brought some barriers, and temptations, but it has also brought some enablers. We can use technology to help us on our weight loss journey. Technology has brought us tools that make it easier to keep to our weight loss goals, such as advances in our nutrition and exercise knowledge through scientific research, and more tangible weight loss enablers like indoor exercise equipment, state of the art kitchen appliances, monitoring programs on mobile devices, information about food products available at our fingertips. We really are more informed than ever.

The problem is most people who try to lose weight go against the flow of change rather than using the momentum to propel them forward. The Good Enough Diet is not only a change in diet and exercise but also a change in mindset!

Be positive about change — use it to your advantage

The more adaptive and flexible you are in life, the more you can thrive in less than ideal situations. When you go with the world, rather than against it, you will be successful not only in losing weight, but in maintaining it as well.

This is the secret of thin people. They know how to live with today. They control their food and the health behaviours they are faced with, rather than letting the changes in the world control them. As food portions get larger, they have more leftovers. As they have more time and less incidental exercise due to technology, they use this time to do more planned exercise. When they are busy, they choose the healthier option when eating out—unless it's a special occasion. Thin people don't blame the world for their problems. Thin people work with the world, and make the best of a bad situation. This is what the Good Enough Diet is about—not getting caught up when you can't control things. Focus instead on how you can respond better to the situation and control what is controllable.

Focus on actions not outcomes

In our clinics people spend a lot of time and energy focusing on the weight they want to be. As you know, concentrating on the outcome rather than the actions to get there can have the opposite effect. The longer you fight with choosing how much weight you want to lose, and how quickly you can do it, the longer you will remain the same. The more time and emotional energy you devote to making a decision like this, the more time and emotional energy you waste that could have been spent on taking a positive approach to your weight loss effort.

The Good Enough Diet isn't a fad diet, therefore it's not a 'wishing diet'. It is a doing diet. Thinking about weight loss takes as much time as actually doing it, so in actual fact it's ineffective to even think about it.

Why we need a new dieting approach

There are a few changes that have been prominent in Australia in the last few decades. The family structure has altered, our working hours have increased and we are travelling more. This is why we have less time, and why we need the Good Enough Diet.

Let's firstly look at the family structure. While nuclear families were the norm up to the 1970s and 1980s, this is not the case today. With more single and blended families, responsibilities and time to focus on diet and exercise are more difficult. Even in many families, both parents now work, so this also adds an extra range of activities that need to be juggled or managed. Before children have reached 14 months old, 45 per cent of mothers have gone back to work.

The nine to five working day is becoming less and less 'normal' for workers in Australia. As we work directly with corporations and businesspeople, we know this is especially true for those who are looking at advancing their career. In 1981, Australia introduced the

38-hour working week, theoretically giving a working Australian adequate time for leisure and sleep per day. Interestingly, in 2006 the ABS report showed that the average Australian worker actually worked 46 hours per week, compared with many other countries averaging less than 43 hours. A quarter of fathers with children under five years of age worked more than 55 hours per week in Australia. We are also taking fewer holidays. Almost 60 per cent of all workers didn't take their annual leave entitlements because they were too busy or were unable to take time off when it suited their needs. The world is different from 1981. Our priorities are different. In a perfect world, we would go back to nine to five, but for the more ambitious in this world, that probably isn't going to cut it if you aim to reach your career or financial goals.

There are many reasons why we are busy. Technology, families, working hours and travelling are just four reasons, but combined they make having a perfect diet and exercise regimen unrealistic. This is why the Good Enough Diet is needed if you want to lose weight without losing your life.

In the following chapters we are going to give you strategies that will allow you to lose weight, even when your life isn't perfect. We're going to show you how our clients who have led busy lives managed to lose weight.

Takeaway tips

- The Good Enough Diet takes into account the changes in technology, family structure, career focus and travel that have occurred in recent years.
- The Good Enough Diet works realistically with today's lifestyles.
- Focus on actions rather than outcomes and you will be successful.
- Forget blaming changes in the world and use them to help you lose weight.
- Control what you can.
- When you can't control a situation, adapt and be as flexible as you can.
- Technology, family, career and travel are great excuses for not losing weight but they are not *reasons* for not losing weight.

Part I GOOD ENOUGH DIET

Chapter 2

PROACTIVE EATING

As health professionals we are used to hearing how external influences affect food choices:

'I was busy at work.'
'I had friends over.'
'There was nothing in the fridge.'
'It was the only thing around.'
'I wasn't feeling very well.'
'I drank too much and was hungry.'
'It was on special.'

These are examples of reactive eating. This happens when you eat something you hadn't planned, and may not even like very much, reactive to the situation you are faced with in the moment.

In the Good Enough Diet, we're not saying that you can't eat treats or junk food, drink alcohol or go out for a nice dinner. What we're saying is that you need to do these on your terms rather than on the terms of food companies, fast-food outlets, emotions, the time available, or influences from friends or family.

Controlling your world to ensure success

Steve Nevitt is the CEO of a large insurance company. His lifestyle consists of long work hours, endless meetings and the occasional confusion of whether he lives in hotel rooms, on aeroplanes or in his home.

This lifestyle is not conducive to losing weight using traditional methods. As much as he would like to, he cannot always plan where he will be too far ahead of schedule. Being in the risk minimisation game, he has tried. However, it is impossible for him to perfectly predict crises or opportunities that will require immediate attention.

Steve was aware that he had a problem. He was aware that his weight had crept up over the years. He was aware that he was in situations where he found it difficult to control his food intake. He was aware that the foods available throughout his working day weren't helping his weight loss efforts. Awareness is the first step in proactive eating, so luckily Steve had part of the battle won.

Steve became aware that he needed help, and that's when he approached us for assistance. Although he was a brilliant problem solver, he couldn't work out how to lose weight with a lifestyle of travel and business commitments, which led to immense frustration with his situation. Steve had challenges that the average person didn't have to face. He worked in Sydney but lived in Melbourne. He travelled interstate at least twice a week and once a quarter he travelled to the US for a week.

Weekly shopping, kilojoule-controlled menus and a regular exercise plan were not going to work for Steve, so we needed to develop a situational plan. We needed to plan for unexpected circumstances so he could get the best results. Sustainable results.

We needed to recruit the stakeholders involved in his life, including his wife, executive assistant and travel companies.

The easiest situation to mark off were meals eaten at home. His wife was very supportive of his weight loss efforts and we gave her options to prepare at home and lists of allowed snacks. She even froze some meals in case there were nights when she was out and Steve had to find his own meals.

We looked at places in the city that served healthy options that he liked to eat and could be delivered to his office. We also looked at other outlets that were within walking distance. We developed 'Steve's Menu' that his executive assistant could order from depending on what he felt like for the day, or what was convenient for him to eat if he had to eat lunch on the run.

Steve was a Qantas platinum frequent flyer, so we looked at the available food in the lounges and on his common flights. We highlighted a heart-healthy, diabetic meal according to his preferences, so he would always be given a healthy choice. Even though he wasn't diabetic or had heart or cholesterol issues, we knew these would be better options for overall weight loss.

For common work travel destinations, we rated hotels according to a healthy hotels system. Because of his gym program, the first priority was to find accommodation with good gym facilities. The second priority was to locate good healthy food options, highlighting the best menu choices that were within walking distance or could be delivered to his hotel. We also looked at the hotel's room service menu and noted the healthy options. We identified where his meetings were and discussed healthy options available if meals or snacks were provided. Once this plan was set in place, we had situations and destinations sorted—for a while anyway. We needed to refine the plan whenever changes to menus occured (we checked these monthly), new outlets opened or we received recommendations from other travellers.

Working with a specific plan and having a support team to assist in the execution and refinement of the plan was the key to Steve's weight loss success. The amount of actual and emotional time devoted to complaining about the difficulty in losing weight if you are busy is huge, whether it be travelling and working away like Steve, or busy ensuring the house is sorted, finances are on track and children are

> *Controlling your world to ensure success (cont'd)*
>
> being chauffeured to their myriad activities. But it needn't be. If this physical and emotional time was diverted to looking for the patterns in your life, you too can make a situational plan. These proactive measures may change every couple of months according to your lifestyle, such as school semesters or other seasonal commitments.

Four stages to proactive eating

You may be excused for thinking that proactive eating is as simple as planning. Yes, planning is important, but planning is not going to help you lose weight. Execution of that plan will. Proactive eating involves four areas — awareness, planning, execution and refinement.

Stage 1: do you really know what you eat?

Being aware of what you eat is the first stage in proactive eating. We make over 200 food and eating decisions every day. What to eat, what type to eat, which brand to eat, how much to eat, when to eat, with whom to eat and so it continues throughout the day. Often we make these decisions reactively, without being aware. We all have little rituals with our food — some are healthy and some are destructive. Many women eat differently at different stages of their menstrual cycle. Many people eat terribly when they travel — even when it is for work and not holidays. Many people go searching for food when they are hungry — often leading to unhealthy choices. Many people fill the cupboards with treats 'for the kids', only to eat them all themselves after a bad day at work. What are your little quirks and rituals? When do you fall down on your diet? Most of the time it will be predictable, and repeated. Knowing what you do in certain situations is helpful. Realising what you are doing when you are doing it is great. Being able to stop when you know you are fuelling emotions rather than hunger is powerful.

Becoming aware of what you are doing and what the triggers are will allow you to set up a plan to overcome this destructive behaviour. Sometimes the reason for your reactive eating may be obvious. Energy-drink-fuelled university students at exam time are an example of this. At other times the obvious reason may not be the actual reason, and may be masking something deeper. We will talk about this in depth in chapter 7, but have you ever thought about why you are sabotaging yourself? What are the benefits for you in being overweight? At first this may seem like a strange question, but a question you should ask yourself nonetheless, and think about it for a while. After all, if there were no benefits for you in being overweight, you wouldn't be overweight — right?

Stage 2: plan to lose weight

Once you have become a little more aware, or at least identified patterns in your eating behaviour, planning is your next step. Planning around your lifestyle is the *only* way you will be able to sustain a healthy eating program.

We have all developed habits and norms from childhood. For example, as children, it is normal and acceptable to eat unhealthily when you travel. However, what we need to realise is that when we travelled as kids, we were going on holiday, and it was at most a few times a year. If your work involves travel or late nights at the office, these situations need to be treated like everyday eating days rather than the exception. As children, we had cake five times a year at home. Christmas cake, of course, and birthday cake for mum's, dad's, our sibling's and our birthdays. Away from the house, a cake surfaced at birthday parties, about every month — on average. It is okay to eat cake on someone's birthday, but when you have an office of hundreds or thousands of colleagues, every day is someone's birthday, and you will need to choose, decide and be proactive about when you eat cake if you want to lose weight.

Planning your food before you have mapped out your life or common situations is useless. We see this all the time with our clients. They plan to exercise or go to the gym without thinking about how they will fit it in. They buy a truckload of fresh fruit and vegetables, only to be out the door three days later on a business trip.

Scenario planning like an athlete

If you can, planning your meals to match the situations you find yourself in is your best option for weight loss. If you know you have a board meeting on a Monday night and you won't get home until 9 pm, having a frozen leftover ready is an example of a situational meal. Athletes do this all of the time to ensure their nutritional intake matches their training and competition schedule. They use their training schedule provided from their coaches, and work with a sports dietitian to match their food to their exercise. Their food changes according to their exercise intensity for their next training session. When you are a businessperson, you need to match your food and nutritional intake with your work, social and family commitments.

If you are unable to plan for exact situations, just like scenario planning in business, at the very least you need to have a best-case, expected-case and worst-case scenario. The best-case scenario is a meal that is prepared and eaten under ideal circumstances. You get home from work with plenty of time to prepare your meal, you were able to do the grocery shopping and you can sit at the dining table to enjoy your nutritious meal. The best-case scenario may be reserved for weekends or quiet times of the year, but when you can do it — do it. The expected-case scenario is the meal that you can eat usually. When you get home from work at the usual time, when you have done some shopping, but there isn't time to get additional forgotten ingredients. These meals may include quick mixed meals, like curries, stir-fries or casseroles. They still include the healthy ingredients within a balanced meal, but may include leftovers, or help from some pre-made ingredients or components. If your day has just not gone to plan, it is time to engage a worst-case scenario option. This may include frozen dinners, frozen leftovers, healthy takeaway or restaurant meals, or something quickly put together. We know you are busy, and like many of our clients before you, the worst-case scenario pops up way more than is ideal, or expected. Chapter 22 is devoted to solutions when you are in this situation.

We don't believe that you need to cut out the foods and drinks you enjoy in life. However, we do emphasise the importance of planning for these.

Can you still treat yourself and lose weight?

When you eat proactively, it's okay to have the occasional treat or alcoholic drink. Again, this needs to be on your terms. The trick is to make an occasion out of treats, rather than allowing them because you're stressed and simply feel you 'deserve them'. This means planning to have an ice cream when you go to the movies with your friends as opposed to sitting at home while reactively eating the whole tub as a result of boredom or a bad day. As a simple rule — eat treats away from the house. This is especially important if you have children too. Instead of having a block of chocolate at home, go out for a chocolate. Instead of having juice or fizzy drinks in the fridge all the time, reserve these for birthdays or drinks with friends. Swap homemade cappuccinos with brewed coffee, and save the milky treat coffee for when you catch up with friends.

Having a planned free meal per week, when you can eat out and have what you choose, will surprisingly help you lose weight in the long run. This is because your diet will not be as restrictive, resulting in rebellion when reactive temptations are too irresistible. Some busy people realise that they will be faced with the worst-case scenario quite often, or may be asked out to dinner at some stage during the week. We don't insist you plan the day and time of your free meal, but keep this flexible. We suggest that when you can eat at your best-case or expected-case scenario, you should take advantage of this. Otherwise, if an invitation falls after your free meal, you will need to be disciplined and choose something diet friendly from the menu on that occasion.

Stage 3: putting it into practice

When planning and execution come together, results are achieved. Creating practical applications of your plan is always helpful. For example, create a shopping list from your weekly menu, create a couple of automatic orders using online shopping services and have worst-case scenario options available for when they are needed.

Usually, if you are too busy to eat well, and you find time and reactive eating a problem, you might also find time to actually make the plan difficult. You know you can plan your healthy eating and exercise situational plan by yourself, but if you know that truthfully you can't do it yourself because of time or other priorities, you may need to enlist health professionals to help you and engage your support team, including family members, your work assistants or others who can make sure your plan is executed well. An accredited practising dietitian (APD) and accredited exercise physiologist (AEP) will be able to ensure that you get on track.

The funny thing about successful people is that they expect to get everything right the first time. We know that we do. The problem is that many of us don't get it right the first time so this why they give up — try something new. You have spent years creating and embedding the food, exercise and eating habits that you have now. They are not going to change instantly after reading this book. They are something you need to continually work on, and when you fail, you have to just take it in your stride as a hiccup, and not give up. It can take months to get the hang of these philosophies and incorporate them into your lifestyle, but it's better to allow yourself time to adjust rather than return to your old ways the next time you fall off the wagon.

Stage 4: changing plans when changing is needed

Once you set a plan, you'll become aware of barriers that you didn't think of before you started. You'll find some unknowing participants that you forgot to account for, like closed food outlets when you planned to use them; cafés that say they deliver but are notoriously late; booked-out hotels; a gift of chocolates from a well-intentioned friend; or additional ingredients that you didn't consider to make the meal you were planning for Friday night.

You will also need to assess your results to ensure that your plan is having the desired outcomes. If not, you may need to make further refinements to achieve your goals.

Your plan will continually need to be refined. You will solve problems that you didn't know existed, and after a few months you will find that it works like clockwork. Like Steve, you need to ensure that you keep your situational plans up to date, and frequently scheduling the updates, as you would your customer database, is imperative to long-term success.

Takeaway tips

- Become aware of situations or environments that result in you reactively eating the wrong foods
- Plan your meals and snacks to match your lifestyle.
- Create a best-case, expected-case and worst-case scenario eating plan.
- Eat treats away from the home. Don't keep them in the house.
- Drink alcohol or other kilojoule-containing drinks away from the home.
- Schedule one 'free meal' per week.
- Enlist a support team to help you achieve your goals.
- Evaluate your results and your plan and make continual refinements until it's perfect.

Chapter 3

THE MAIN INGREDIENT

If you want to lose weight, no amount of special pills, potions or fancy foods will help you more than the main ingredient. Albeit boring, if you want to lose weight, the easiest way is to eat more of the main diet ingredient — non-starchy vegetables. The more of these you eat, the more weight you will be able to lose. Over the years, there have been fad diets that say you can't put on weight by eating too much of different foods or nutrients — low-fat diets preached that you couldn't get fat from eating too many carbohydrates. Low-carbohydrate diets preached that you couldn't get fat from eating too much protein or fat, as long as the carbohydrate is low. Low-sugar, or low-fructose, diets preach that the only thing that makes you fat is sugar, and particularly the sugar found in fruit. Sadly, we know that none of these claims are true. The claims sound easy, they sound sexy, they sound reassuring, they sound too good to be true — and they are. Carbohydrates, protein and fat are all needed for different functions in the body. Eating too little of any of these nutrients will cause you health problems, while eating too much of any of these nutrients will cause you to put on weight.

What's the non-negotiable in weight loss?

The truth is that to lose weight, non-starchy vegetables need to be the focus of your diet. Being low in kilojoules, high in vitamins and minerals, and high in fibre make non-starchy vegetables a perfect diet food. Vegetables unlock fuel for the cells, help you feel full and cut down the overall kilojoules of a meal. For a full list of non-starchy vegetables, see appendix A.

You wouldn't find a health professional that didn't agree with this, but getting you to eat them is a little harder. If you have just started reading this book and you haven't completed all of the components of the diet just yet, if you take away one thing—remember this—non-starchy vegetables are the key to your weight loss success. The Good Enough Diet proves that if you eat non-starchy vegetables in all of your meals, you will lose weight.

Tim Brackenridge — vegetable skeptic

'Hmmm, I don't eat vegetables', said Tim, looking at Tara like he was the one being called into the principal's office. 'Okay, so this part is not negotiable', Tara responded, almost taking on the role of the principal. 'It's just like school attendance—some of the kids don't like it, but they still have to do it—we'll train you to do it.'

Tim Brackenridge is a senior secondary school principal, with over 150 teachers and 2000 students. Busy with meetings that come with the territory of running a new large school while trying to be a good dad and husband resulted in Tim's health taking a back seat. Lunchtime was filled with student meetings, after school was filled with teacher meetings, and consequently meals were rare and usually something quick with little nutritional value.

In these situations, it's common to see a family with similar health profiles, but not in Tim's case. His slim wife and fit 18-year-old son had been nagging him to eat well, just like when Tim was a maths teacher, nagging the kids to make sure their homework was completed.

Tim first met Tara at a presentation she did for secondary school principals. He reluctantly decided to make an appointment with her, knowing the types of things she was going to say, and the fact that he probably wouldn't like what she was going to suggest.

Tim had tried many fad diets in the past, but although he lost weight in the short term, as soon as he returned to his hectic life his weight went straight back on.

'The problem is quite simple — I just don't like vegetables', Tim revealed. Tara listened, but to be honest, it wasn't the first time she had heard 'I don't like x, y or z'.

'What if there is no such thing as taste?' Tara asked. Being a science teacher, Tim thought he was about to be tricked and had reservations about taking this point of view without putting up a fight.

Tara and Tim discussed her theory that taste is merely perception, and if it is perception it could be challenged and changed.

For Tim, we used the laddering approach to creating familiarity and therefore acceptance of a variety of vegetables. We started with one vegetable at a time, ensuring that the food was introduced in a good environment with a positive attitude. We introduced each vegetable at half a serve a time and prepared it in different ways.

By introducing walking after school as his third space (which will be discussed in more detail in chapter 16) and simply making vegetables feature in his diet, Tim went from almost 110 kilograms to a trim 87 kilograms in a few months. His waist measurement reduced from 124 centimetres to 100 centimetres, putting him at much lower risk of heart disease, type 2 diabetes and, most importantly, nagging from his fitness-focused family.

For Tim, just two little strategies that could fit easily into his life resulted in almost 25 kilograms of weight loss, and major improvements to his health and longevity. By just adding non-starchy vegetables to his meals, Tim's diet became good enough to lose weight.

The truth about taste

The truth is taste preferences are more about other factors than the actual sensations emitted by our taste buds in response to different foods. Taste preferences are simply perceptions, beliefs and habits developed in early childhood, but they do change over time and with intervention.

Familiarity is the biggest contributor to taste preferences. It's why Australians love Vegemite, why Thai children will eat Thai curries but not Indian curries, and why Asians enjoy a variety of seafood. If you travel frequently and move between different cultures, you'll find that you start to enjoy a variety of foods, even ones you initially found confronting, but you can also sample these cuisines at home and develop a taste for food outside your comfort zone.

Strategies to change taste are not an overnight occurrence — although they can be. When you have grown up not liking a food, you will continue to have negative associations with that food.

It is known that new taste buds take at least three weeks to develop, but the psychological aspect of changing taste preferences can take much longer. In children, it has been shown that they need to be exposed to a new food more than 11 times before they will accept it. Funnily enough, we have tried this with numerous adults, and the same is true.

You can introduce a variety of healthy foods and train yourself to like them. You can also do this for big kids, like husbands or teenagers who refuse to make changes to their diet.

The first stage is to try the new vegetable in a mixed meal, such as grated in pasta sauces, or cut small in stir-fries or curries. Especially if the dish contains strong flavours and smells, there is no way you'll taste the new vegetable, although those adamant not to change will argue otherwise.

The same vegetable needs to be included three different ways in meals that are not mixed, aiming for at least three times per week. For example, try broccoli mixed through pasta, served steamed from the microwave alongside your regular vegetables, or steamed and then mixed into a stir-fry.

You only need to eat small amounts to change your taste preferences. Although a bite of broccoli might not improve your nutritional intake remarkably at first, the benefits to familiarity and long-term acceptance are worth it. This can also go the other way. For example, for children, a tiny sip of soft drink or a finger dipped into chocolate spread may not negatively affect their nutritional intake, but can be the start of poor taste preferences for the child who becomes a teenager who becomes an adult.

Creating a positive environment for different foods that you once didn't like is needed to create positive associations with new foods. Use simple strategies such as self-suggesting ('I love...prepared this way'), and make sure you eat in a calm environment without negative distractions or fights. This is why arguing with children about eating certain foods only exacerbates distaste for certain foods.

At the start, this is something you have to make yourself do. Challenge yourself. Once you challenge yourself, it will become habit and sooner or later, like Tim, you'll be saying, 'Do you remember when I didn't eat that?'

Any time is the right time

Sitting in a café eating breakfast in Thailand, Adam started to write. He saw first-hand something interesting that he and Tara had been discussing when forming this book. It was interesting to see what the Thai locals ate for breakfast. Cereal? Toast? Fruit? Yoghurt? — no! Breakfast foods were the same as lunch and dinner foods — stir-fries. Yes, many Asian cultures include vegetables at breakfast, mostly fish or meat and vegetables with rice; however, this is seen as strange in Western cultures. Western cultures create norms that, like taste, are more psychologically relevant than nutritionally important, such as the Australian standard of Vegemite on toast or the American breakfast of hot pancakes and maple syrup.

If you can include vegetables at breakfast, this will be a great start to ensuring you get your vegetable requirements for the day. And having some additional nutrients with breakfast is so important for a busy worker.

You don't need to eat stir-fries or salads for breakfast, but there are still plenty of ways to include vegetables at this meal:

- tomato and avocado on wholegrain toast
- roasted mushrooms, tomatoes, asparagus and capsicum on wholegrain toast
- low-fat ricotta, spinach, tomato and smoked salmon on wholegrain toast

- low-fat cottage cheese, capsicum, eggplant and onion on wholegrain toast
- ratatouille and poached eggs
- spinach savoury pancakes (great for St Patrick's day!)
- vegetable omelette.

Preparing tasty vegetables

Many people don't eat, and think they don't like, some vegetables because they don't know how to prepare them. Again, this comes down to familiarity rather than true taste preferences. It's traditional in our Western culture to eat meals of meat and three vegetables, but you don't need to stick to rules like this.

Using flavourings such as garlic, ginger, herbs and spices can make vegetables tastier, and make a dish taste completely different from the night before. Adding vegetables to all mixed meals, or eating a dish with vegetables or a salad on the side, is a good way to keep your vegetable intake high and your kilojoule intake low.

A salad or vegetables can be interchangeable, but make sure you choose your ingredients from the non-starchy vegetable list (see appendix A) because salad additions like eggs, bacon, cheese, oily or creamy sauces and croutons aren't vegetables — or salads.

For other types of foods, which will be discussed in later chapters, we suggest you limit the variety of foods within food groups, and that you serve them directly onto your plate rather than from a dish in the middle of the table, as this results in overeating. With non-starchy vegetables, we suggest you serve some with your main meal and leave some in a dish on the centre of the table, which will encourage you and your family to take extra servings.

Preparing vegetables in a variety of ways is the key to keeping you and your family interested in including them with each meal. However, for some people, it's not the variety of preparation techniques that is the problem, it's the lack of convenience.

Making vegetables convenient

We know that vegetables and salads take time to prepare; they are perishable, last for only a few days and can mean more trips to the supermarket or farmers market.

If you don't have time, the next option is to use frozen vegetables. These are easily thrown into mixed meals or steamed in the microwave. Frozen vegetables don't need to be cooked in water as they will go soggy; however, they still have a similar texture to fresh vegetables when cooked. Frozen vegetables have continually been proven to hold the same nutritional content of fresh vegetables, so although they are easier to prepare, you're not compromising on nutrients. Just be sure to get a variety of types, and choose mostly non-starchy frozen varieties.

How much is enough?

As Marjorie Dawes tells us in *Little Britain*, 'Just take what you're eating and cut it in half'.

Doing one simple thing will drop your weight easily without too much thought or effort on your behalf. This simple thing is making sure half of your plate is made up of non-starchy vegetables. The more of your meal that is made up of non-starchy vegetables, the better your weight loss results will be. Using this simple strategy, in a research study a group of overweight Canadians with diabetes lost significantly more weight, had greater reductions in cholesterol and better blood sugar results than a control group who followed standard nutritional guidelines.

The current National Health and Medical Research Council (NHMRC) dietary guidelines for all Australians suggest that you should eat five serves of vegetables per day. One serve is one cup of salad, or half a cup of vegetables. This is not too hard to reach, but instead of focusing on how many serves you're having, try to increase the amount of non-starchy vegetables you eat and continually look for opportunities to add them to your meals and overall diet.

Non-starchy vegetables are also great to keep in the fridge to snack on while you are starting on your lower kilojoule eating plan. Green beans, cherry tomatoes, snow peas, baby cucumbers and baby carrots all make wonderful already prepared convenience foods. You can also cut up other vegetables and store in a container for when you want a snack on the go — broccoli, cauliflower, celery and capsicum make delicious cool, fresh snacks.

When eating out, or ordering takeaway, always ask for additional vegetables or a side salad if they are available.

Takeaway tips

- Eating non-starchy vegetables is the key to losing weight and gaining health.
- Eat non-starchy vegetables with all meals.
- Fill half your plate with non-starchy vegetables or salad.
- Keep a range of non-starchy vegetables in the fridge for you to snack on.
- Always keep frozen vegetables in the freezer in case of emergencies.
- Remember, taste is more about familiarity than actual taste.
- If you don't like a vegetable, you will need to try it more than 11 times before you will accept or like it.
- Even if the recipe doesn't call for it, add more non-starchy vegetables.

Chapter 4

VARIETY

They say variety is the spice of life — but variety may be adding a little more sugar than spice to our waistlines.

As you flip through diet books or browse healthy meal plans in magazines or on the internet, you'll notice that most contain a large variety of different foods and meals. You will be offered a different breakfast every day, different snacks, different lunches and different dinners. The menus provided are weekly, monthly or three-monthly plans promising that you won't get bored and therefore the diets will be sustainable.

But could this be one of the diet industry's biggest failings? After all, although we know they're not healthy, isn't it interesting that fad diets, which shed weight quickly, allow a limited variety of food? Isn't it interesting that when you talk to health professionals, such as doctors, dietitians or exercise physiologists, they commonly profess to eating a low variety of foods for meals — particularly breakfasts and lunch meals?

Is eating a variety of foods aiding our insatiable appetites for different foods, different tastes and different experiences? Or is eating a variety of foods leading us to overeat, or become overwhelmed with making a choice, and taking us back to the unhealthy habits formed in the past when we ate what we wanted to and didn't have to think about it?

When we consider the perfect level of variety, in the Good Enough Diet we should aim for somewhere in the middle of the no variety presented by many fad diets to the highly varied menus presented by many *healthy* eating plans.

I'll have 'the usual'

It's a normal Wednesday morning at the Tanner household. After eating her usual breakfast, Jules is preparing the family's lunches, as well as her own. As a single mum of three, Jules has lots to think about and do. She is finishing her nursing degree while working part time at a local aged-care facility. Luckily, healthy breakfasts and lunches are something she doesn't have to worry about—she just makes 'the usual'—and they can be sorted quickly and easily, without giving them a second thought.

Jules' weight had skyrocketed to 130 kilograms after her husband's unforeseen passing from a sudden heart attack at 40 years old, and her son's diagnosis of autism. She had so much on her plate, and just didn't have the time, energy or mental space to be perfect.

When she was diagnosed with type 2 diabetes, Jules decided she needed to do something about her weight. After three months, her weight had reduced to 118 kilograms, Jules' life was completely changed; she had lost a lot of weight, but not a huge amount considering how much she still had to go. She loved exercising and eating healthily, but after this initial phase she realised that the priorities of her children, her study and her work remained. How could she fit in her newfound love of exercise and desire for weight loss while still being a fabulous mum, committed student and hard worker?

Each time Jules had tried to lose weight, she was given a complicated menu plan. Even her home-delivered meals, which were different each day, still required her to have think about how and where she would eat. She found the emotional time she spent on her diet was severely affecting the time she had available for other things. Something had to give to help Jules continue to lose weight, and we decided it was going to be variety.

Together, Jules and Tara developed a meal plan that offered the same breakfast on most days — porridge; the same snacks — fruit, yoghurt or nuts; the same lunch — mountain bread with cottage cheese, cucumber and red capsicum or a salad wrap with tinned fish or chicken; and the same dinner — chicken, salmon, pork or beef with steamed vegetables and a carbohydrate choice, such as rice, pasta or potato.

Jules found this low level of variety good enough to lose weight. She continued on the diet for seven more months and her weight continued to drop to 90 kilograms. Her goal weight was 82 kilograms, so we didn't have much further to go. Even after Jules' weight was stabilising, she continued to stick to low variety for her breakfast and lunch meals. If you were in Jules' kitchen right now while she was preparing her family's lunch, you'd notice that the kids got sandwiches, and she would have salmon, some salad and a slice of wholegrain bread. Her breakfast dishes in the sink would contain the remnants of her porridge and her children's cereal and milk. It doesn't matter whether you were watching her last week, today or in a month. Breakfast and lunch would be the same.

'It is just so much easier to keep my weight in check if I eat the same food every day', shares Jules. 'We often change what goes into the kids' sandwiches and occasionally I will have chicken or ham instead of salmon, but it pretty much stays the same.'

Jules finds this routine positive for her weight loss as well as her stress levels. 'What we have for lunch and breakfast is just something that we don't need to think about. It's like having the kids in school uniform, and me in my work uniform ... choosing the kids' school clothes would be a constant battle in the morning.'

> *I'll have 'the usual' (cont'd)*
>
> 'I like variety, but we have different dinners. If I'm eating out or at mum's we will eat what she has prepared, if we're at home it's the same.' Keeping to similar foods every day has made meal preparation, shopping and keeping within budget much easier. Surprisingly, Jules finds it easier to stick to this diet than an elaborate plan. 'Interestingly, not only do I not mind keeping my meals the same, I find it less boring than if I changed daily. I get variety fatigue when I introduce new foods for a while, and often go back to my usual.'
>
> Jules reached her goal weight and has maintained it for over 12 months now. She continues to be as active as she can. Now she has finished her study and is working as a nurse. She continues to eat the same breakfast, and has organised meals at work to be similar to what she would prepare for herself at home.

Do you really need variety?

Diets are written in one of two directions. Many have a completely different option suggested for each meal, changing every day. Alternatively they cut out whole food groups, or have food types that are not allowed, resulting in people eating quite a bland and unbalanced diet.

Although a varied diet plan may be perfectly developed to align with dietary guidelines and maximise nutrient intake, it might not be very user-friendly. Eating different foods every day means that your fridge and pantry needs to be full so you have the ingredients available to make the suggested meals. This can mean that a lot food is wasted if it isn't used by its expiry date or if fresh foods become old and wilted. Leftovers won't be eaten, which leads to increased waste. Full fridges and pantries with a variety of foods are also not ideal for those who suffer from emotional or binge eating. The less food variety available, the less food will be eaten.

To plan three new meals per day (or more with snacks) can take a lot of effort. When you're already thinking about work, home and recreation, planning different meals and making sure you have the ingredients can take up a lot of emotional space.

The funny thing is that if you consider those who have been successful at losing weight, like Jules, they will tell you that they eat a relatively *boring* diet. They eat the same foods often and some proclaim that they have eaten the same food every day for the past 5, 10, 15 or 20 years.

As health professionals we have both been guilty of eating one way and prescribing another in the past as well. Adam eats exactly the same breakfast, bircher muesli, and exactly the same lunch, tinned fish, salad and bread, every day when he is home. Tara eats the same breakfast, and switches after a few weeks to something different until the next change in a few weeks' time. For example, one week may be baked beans on toast, the next porridge and the next poached eggs on a nine-grain bread or a fruit English muffin. Living by herself, she cooks meals like fish and vegetable curries, or chicken and vegetable stir-fries, that make three to four serves. One serve will cover the meal she is eating, with enough leftovers for the next day or two's lunches and dinners, meaning no cooking for a couple of days. Although it's important that your meal plan suits your lifestyle, we have provided some ideas in appendix C to give you a head start.

Despite the fact that we don't get bored with what we are eating, we were both taught to always prescribe something new for our clients who were trying to lose weight. But our attitude changed when we realised that less variety equals more weight loss.

Less variety equals *more* weight loss

After a few years of prescribing diets with varied meals, we realised that this commonly used strategy to help people lose weight was flawed. It was flawed for a number of reasons, and the patterns became glaringly obvious after a few significant events.

Firstly we became aware that our research data continually agreed with a study released almost 10 years ago from Tufts University and the National Weight Control Registry in the US. They found that those who lost weight and kept it off for more than two years had less variety within all food groups except vegetables, and more variety in their choice of vegetables. This meant that they were not cutting out food groups, but having less of a variety within each of them. More recently, Dr Leonard Epstein and his team of researchers at the University at Buffalo have been studying how variety affects children's eating behaviours and childhood obesity. His 12 experiments published in 2009 and 2010 found that increasing variety was the best way to increase food intake and therefore weight in children. Interestingly, they also discovered that increasing the variety of exercise types could increase the amount of exercise that children did. Maybe this would work for you too?

We next analysed our clients and came to realise that we could group them into two types: those whom we would give full meal plans or books that ensured their meals varied each day, and those whom we would give example meal plans based on the healthy food they liked with limited variation.

Against logic, those with *more* variety would proclaim 'I'm bored' far more often than those who were given *less* variety. Those with less variety were rigid about changing, and we would hear comments such as 'Can't I just keep having x, y, z for lunch? I really like it' or 'I just find it easier to eat that every day' and 'When I have had enough of that, or stop losing weight, I will change'. The most common responses used to describe the non-varied diet were that it was 'easy', 'achievable', 'habit forming' and 'easy' (because it was said twice as often as the rest).

More variety equals more food

As well as making weight loss easier and taking up less mental energy, less variety also means consuming less food. Usually when you eat at home, having one plate of food is fine. You are satisfied. You are full. You are happy.

If you are at a buffet or there is a big spread of food with lots of choice, say, on Christmas day, you tend to eat more than you need. It's easy to suffer from smorgasbord syndrome when you can choose a little bit of this and a little bit of that. If you have only one plate you feel dissatisfied or deprived. You feel hungry. You're not happy with just one plate. If there is dessert, and two options, it's tempting to have a little bit of everything.

So, it's pretty simple. If you want to eat less of something or less of a type of food, have less variety available. This means if you want a treat food, only have one type available. If you need to eat less carbohydrates at night, don't serve a curry that includes potato on a bed of rice, accompanied by bread. Choose one of the carbohydrates — rice, bread or potatoes. If you want to eat more of something, have more variety available. As we discussed in chapter 3, have plenty of non-starchy vegetables available, so even if part of your meal is not as healthy as it could be, you can reduce the overall damage by having less kilojoule-laden food and more nutrient-dense, low-kilojoule food.

Takeaway tips

- Don't be pressured into varying your meals too often.
- Eat similar meals at your busiest time in the day.
- Don't go grocery shopping when you're hungry.
- Offer one option of kilojoule-containing foods. For example, have one protein (meat, chicken or fish) and one carbohydrate option (potato, rice, pasta or noodles).
- Offer a bigger variety of non-starchy vegetables. This means you will eat more of these low-kilojoule foods.
- When you eat out, plan what you will eat before you go, or when you arrive. This will keep you from eating reactively to what looks good.
- Breakfast is the easiest meal to keep stable. You can eat the same thing daily, or you can vary weekly.
- Buy only what you need. Smorgasbord syndrome can also be 'supermarket syndrome'.
- Always keep at least one food consistent if you're packing lunches for children.
- Serve up meals rather than having people serve their own.

Chapter 5

COMFORT FOOD

Unfortunately, food plays a much bigger role in our lives than just being nourishment for our bodies. Dietitians often use the analogy of food being like fuel for a car: you wouldn't put low-grade fuel into a high-performance car, so why put low-grade fuel into the high-performance machine that is your body? If only it were that simple. If only cars had social and emotional needs, maybe the analogy would be a little more accurate.

For some people, emotional eating and positive associations beyond taste are not a problem. For these people, the concept of proactive eating is simple. If it's good for me, I'll eat it — if not I'll just have a small bit, occasionally, or in moderation. However, for others the psychological, emotional and social connection to food is stronger than any physical need or want.

In society — not just today, but historically — food is involved in celebrations and commiserations, as well as mundane events like meetings. It brings together families, cultures and teams, and when good food is present, the smiles that beam across faces highlight the importance of it in our world.

Having a positive relationship towards food doesn't mean that all emotional connections need to be severed, but the ones that bring about guilt and other feelings that are not helpful for our wellbeing are best to be managed if we want to achieve good enough weight loss.

It starts at an early age

Tara, co-author of this book, battled with her weight throughout childhood—probably one of the reasons she became a dietitian. One situation sticks with her more than any others from childhood. Tara spent her first seven years in an Indigenous community in the Kimberley region in Western Australia. Generally a happy child, she had one love—food. At the age of four, Tara was a little chubby, so her mum, Diane, took her to see the visiting dietitian.

Malnutrition and failure to thrive were rife among the Aboriginal kids in Indigenous communities, and these were the dietitian's usual cases. Julie, the dietitian, was friendly enough, and she talked to Diane about what needed to change in Tara's diet to get her weight back to a healthy level. One of the suggestions—and the only one Tara can remember—was no more ice-cream cones from the pre-school canteen. The ice-cream was a strategy introduced to give the malnourished kids some extra kilojoules to increase their weight, and it was working well for that purpose. However, for the chubby kids, it was not the best approach. Every day for a couple of weeks, Tara would line up to get her ice-cream, only to be told by the canteen lady that she wasn't allowed one. For a four year old this was hard to understand, but Diane continued to reassure Tara that it wasn't because she was naughty, just because ice-cream was a treat and not an everyday food.

A few months later, school holidays began and the Diversi family headed to visit Nan and Pop Diversi in Cairns—the big city! Tara doesn't remember the 26 hours of driving to get there in the scalding desert heat. The family travelled in the metallic brown Toyota Corolla that her dad had bought her mum as a gift when Tara was born.

Air-conditioning was a rare luxury, one that the Diversi family didn't have, and you can just imagine the joy of entertaining two kids under six, 25 years ago, before all of the technologies we enjoy today. One thing about that trip that Tara will never forget was the visit to the Woree Drive-In. Could she remember the movie she saw? No. Who else was there? No idea. The only thing she remembered was her choc top ice-cream—every detail from the red-brick kiosk that sold them, the crinkle of the plastic packet, to the crunch of the chocolate topping, the smooth creamy taste of the vanilla ice-cream through to the soggy yellowish cone. Now this was happiness right there.

To this day, if you go with or see Tara at the movies, more than 25 years later, she will eat a choc top ice-cream, and regardless of her mood, whether she is already happy, sad or feeling fat—the joy that comes with the crinkling of the plastic wrap will light up the cinema, just like it did years ago.

This is an example of a long-term connection to food. Today choc top ice-creams are not a connoisseur's choice of ice-cream or dessert. From the fake chocolate topping, the super-hard ice-cream through to the soggy cone, it's not something a food lover would rate as quality. But it is not the taste that continues the purchase over other options, it's the emotional connection that was formed and embedded since childhood.

Emotional eating

Contrary to popular belief, emotional eating doesn't just affect middle-aged women. Those who seek our advice about it vary from children to older adults and seem to be an equal mix of men and women. Most people emotionally eat at some stage or another.

History has long associated food with love. We prepare loved ones meals, and to celebrate success, or to cure pain, we provide food, including treats and sweets.

A continual association of feelings towards treat or junk foods helps us to create emotional connections to food. If you were given chocolate every time you hurt yourself as a child, as an adult the pain caused by a broken heart, boredom, anger or a bad day at work will also feel as though it can be cured with chocolate. If your true family connection was signified by a Sunday roast, missing your family will call for a roast meal.

Not all connections are destructive, and it's worth choosing your battles, and accepting some of the emotional connections, like Tara's choc tops, as just an interesting quirk. However, if you have too many of these, you're using food (or alcohol) as medication or connections needed to be fulfilled daily, which is when problems can start to arise.

Being aware of the emotions that cause you to overeat or to eat junk food is important. Some things that cure emotional eating in one person may exacerbate the feelings that lead another person to emotionally eat in the first place. For example, for one person, a massage is the ultimate stress relief and relaxer—for others, it can seem like an added stressor because it is taking up valuable time or may trigger painful emotions because of the constant physical touch.

Life is very difficult to control, as are our feelings that accompany life. However, food is not. Food is commonly used to regain a sense of control, particularly when life seems to be spiralling out of control.

Guilt often follows emotional eating, and when you emotionally eat, the pain caused by guilt is a trade-off for the feeling you want to suppress, whether it is depression, boredom, rejection, loneliness or anger. When you emotionally eat, take notice of the emotion you're trying to suppress and take the time to get used to feeling this emotion. Just like food, the more familiar you become with the emotion, the more you will be able to accept it and cope with feeling that way.

Eating emotionally occasionally is not a huge issue; however, if it's starting to affect your weight and wellbeing, finding another strategy to improve your mood is the cure. If your emotions are associated with clinical issues such as depression or anxiety, getting professional help for these issues is important, and even if these emotions are not directly associated with your weight, you may find that addressing your problem will result in weight loss.

Accepting that you may not always win against emotional eating is helpful. If you're feeling very reactive, you need to calm down to get back into a positive and proactive mindset. If you find your heart racing and that you're breathing very quickly, you need to slow your breathing to stop the reaction. Sitting down and taking three to seven slow, deep breaths can help you think more proactively rather than reactively.

Internal negotiation

We negotiate with ourselves constantly, and often an episode of emotional overeating follows a negotiation. You are much more likely to positively win the negotiation if it is spoken out loud or written down, so you have time to proactively note and correct the self-sabotage. Otherwise, much of the negotiation is simply justification. You can also come to a compromise. Negotiate with yourself to delay the overeating episode after a period of time (such as 20 minutes), an activity (walk around the block, a warm shower) or making yourself a hot drink, like a cup of tea. If the feeling does not pass, it will at least reduce.

The following suggestions are a guide only. Emotional eating is extremely complex, and some of the techniques discussed might not work for you all the time. However, if they reduce the amount you eat and the frequency of your overeating, you will be able to manage your emotional eating.

Understand that we all have issues

Eating is just one way to cope with our emotions. People engage in numerous other forms of destructive (violence, alcohol) or constructive (exercise, reading) self-medication to manage their emotions. The more you identify with being an emotional eater — 'I'm an emotional eater' — the harder it will be for you to break the cycle. In chapter 14 we discuss how to change this mindset in more detail, but simply changing how you talk to others and yourself about how you cope with these emotions, the better your weight loss efforts will be. For example, it is easy to positively change your story: 'When I'm sad, I play my favourite music to cheer me up', 'When I'm exhausted, I drink some water to get my energy levels back up', 'When I'm bored, I finish off the jobs I've been procrastinating about' or 'When I feel fat, I make myself see my strengths'.

Just because someone is thin and/or beautiful, doesn't mean that they don't have any emotional issues. We all have issues. Some of us wear these issues on the inside and some of us wear them on the outside. The difficulty when you are overweight is that people make assumptions that might not be correct, and it is much easier to notice one issue — a weight issue.

Healthy comfort foods

If you're a heavy eater, that is, you like big portions and you feel you can never be filled, a strategy to help you feel full is to eat more warm meals. In fact, some of our clients benefit from eating only warm cooked meals if they are the type of person who tends to overeat. You'll know if you are one of these people — it can be heard in statements like 'I didn't have any breakfast, I only had some fruit' or 'I'm starving, I only had a salad'.

In 2010 we attended the National Speakers Association's annual convention in Orlando, Florida. Now, a group of speakers who live out of hotel rooms and on aeroplanes could probably do with, and should be grateful for, the occasional healthy meal. On day two of the conference, out came lunch. Screwed-up noses followed the meals being delivered, like a Mexican wave. We were a bit frightened about what we were going to receive, but truly delighted when salad was presented to us. The salad wasn't a plain non-starchy vegetable salad, mind you. It included two types of cheese, two types of meat — chicken and ham — as well as an egg. It was a substantial meal. That day, the wails about how starving everyone was because of lunch overwhelmed the learning from the brilliant speakers. The salad even got a mention in the treasurer's report on the final day, accompanied by a roar of laughter signifying agreement to the perception that a side dish was presented as a meal. The kilojoules in the salad made it enough for a meal, and we were sure that no one was truly physically hungry. But does that matter? No. People were still mentally hungry.

Brain versus belly hunger

Mental hunger is different from physical hunger because regardless of what your body is saying, your head still says you're hungry. Some health professionals suggest that if you're hungry have a piece of fruit, and if you don't want that, then you're not truly hungry. Oh, if it were only this simple. Truth is, you might still be mentally hungry after having a piece of fruit anyway, and end up eating extra later.

Warm food is a great comfort as it reduces mental hunger much more effectively than cold food. If you can have cooked meals or warm snacks, you will have a much better chance of curbing your hunger. For example, if you find that the period after work is a weakness for you and your mouth is like a human vacuum cleaner as soon as you walk in the door, it may be best to plan a warm snack in advance. Some of our clients find success by drinking a warm cup of tea. Others need something a bit heartier, and a warm cup of soup or a bowl of vegetable soup that was frozen in individual packets does the trick perfectly. Other options include steamed vegetables with warmed leftover lean meat, chicken or fish, or a similar mini meal. Eating warm lunches (of course, with plenty of non-starchy vegetables) and warm breakfasts as well as the usual warm dinner meals may allow you to better control your *hunger* and mental hunger.

Reducing sweet comforts

Women in particular are prone to eating sweet comfort foods and snacks. There are many reasons for this, but it seems to be more a mental craving than a physical one. If it were a physical craving, healthier sweet substitutes such as fruit instead of chocolate would do the trick. We all know that this doesn't happen often.

If this is an occasional occurrence, it isn't a huge problem and might not need addressing. So how do you define occasional versus regular? Well, if you crave chocolate on the first day of your menstrual cycle and have a small chocolate bar to compensate, this is probably okay. On average, one sweet comfort a month is not an issue. However, if you crave and satisfy your craving for the week or so of your pre-menstrual and menstrual cycle, this is too much compensation. One week in an average month is too much.

Sometimes sweet cravings can be in response to changing hormone levels, and therefore a diet that evens your blood sugar and hormone levels will be a better option than the band-aid solution of eating the sweet food. This means eating a diet with more protein in the morning, and a low glycaemic index carbohydrate if you're getting those cravings at 3.30 pm.

Supplements such as chromium may be helpful for some women, particularly women with type 2 diabetes, pre-diabetes, polycystic ovarian syndrome and high insulin levels. However, in our experience, those who are strongly affected by food preoccupation and food cravings achieve better results when they work on their mental attitude towards cravings rather than the physical reasons for cravings.

For many, cravings are a normal part of life and a normal feeling that is reactive to a particular situation. Reducing the likelihood of cravings involves ensuring there are no highly craved foods close to you at home or at the office. This is one of the reasons we suggest you only eat treats away from home. Once your environment is a treat-free zone, don't expect to never be hit by that insatiable craving again. The first stage in managing cravings is to accept that this feeling is normal, and having cravings is not good or bad — just part of life. Although satisfying the craving is the easiest option and this may cure the feeling at the time, it will increase the intensity of an unsatisfied craving later on. You need to be open to the fact that you cannot control how you feel, but you can control how you act on this feeling. Relax, take a few deep breaths and allow your proactive self to come back into the equation. After a few months of actively being able to feel one way and act another will bring power, but also a sense of calm when you develop cravings again. Saying out loud to yourself 'I can't control how I feel, I can control how I behave' is a good way to help you cope with cravings. It can also be reassuring to know you have a scheduled treat or free meal coming up in the near future.

Takeaway tips

- Recognise the origin of your comfort foods.
- Determine which of your comfort foods you need to reduce, and which ones are okay.
- Identify some of the positive reasons for being overweight and how you may be self-sabotaging.
- Accept that you will have cravings for different foods.
- Take power in the fact that you don't need to act on cravings.
    - When you are negotiating with yourself, compromise for a win–win situation.
    - When you are anxious, take three deep breaths and calm down before making a decision.
    - Before emotional eating, wait 20 minutes to delay the feeling.
- Create diversions to add time between eating comfort foods.
- Eat warm foods and meals.
- Don't have treats close to you at home or at work.

Chapter 6

IS LOW-FAT FOOD MAKING YOU FAT?

We hate to admit it, but part of our preparation for this book was scoping out the supermarkets and skimming other shoppers' trolleys as we looked for patterns in how everyday Australians eat. We went to large supermarkets, farmers markets, upscale delis and 'healthfood' stores. What we found amazing was the number of shoppers who choose low-fat or diet products. What is even more amazing is that they looked at labels, compared them and in the end chose the low-fat product. When we checked the product after they had moved on, there was very little difference in kilojoule content. We heard more and more people asking attendants for healthy alternatives, and flashes of pride sweeping the faces of those who chose the seemingly healthier alternative. So, in such a health-conscious society, why are we continuing to gain weight at a rate that is out of control? Considering the facts, it could be possible that low-fat food is making us fat.

Eating low-fat food is always highlighted as being the healthiest choice, but in countries such as France where heart disease and diabetes are not yet a significant problem, low-fat products are practically non-existent. In Australia and other countries like the US where obesity and other lifestyle diseases are at an all-time high, almost every product has a low-fat or 'diet' alternative.

But it's low-fat

'But they are low-fat', said Janelle, justifying her daily blueberry muffin for morning tea, and 50 grams of rice crackers for afternoon tea that appeared frequently in her food diary.

Janelle Croker is a baby boomer, working as an executive assistant to a CEO of a Fortune 500 company, a position she is proud to have held for 18 years. Her two children are grown up—Alex, a successful chartered accountant, and Krystal, finishing off her final year at university to qualify as a registered nurse. She enjoys looking after her family and her boss, to make sure they achieve all the success she feels they deserve. However, years of looking after others has meant she has neglected her own health for some time, her weight escalating to 83 kilograms and developing type 2 diabetes.

The issue with Janelle's diet is not just what she eats, but the fact that she thinks what she is eating is healthy diet food. Over the years, she has been on many diet programs, but what she has learnt is that you can eat as much of what you like as long as it's low-fat.

On inspecting her cupboards, we discovered that she has low-fat cereal, low-fat crackers, low-fat snacks and even low-fat *lollies*. No wonder she has put on 20 kilograms over the past six years.

'I just thought it was healthy for me. I was excited that the low-fat labels on the packaging made it so much easier for me to make healthier choices at the supermarket now', said Janelle.

When we went to the supermarket, Janelle was amazed to see that the foods she thought were healthier contained about the same kilojoules as the original, or just a little bit better. Added to the fact that Janelle often justifed her second helpings or second snacks with 'but it's low-fat', she was actually eating much more than she would have if she'd chosen the full-fat or regular version. Being low-fat was one of the biggest reactive eating traits of Janelle's diet plan. She was never

> tempted by the unhealthy treats that made regular appearances in her office, but as soon as someone would say 'but it's low-fat', she found the food hard to resist. Low-fat food was making Janelle fat.

The lowdown on low-fat

Although low-fat products have the same amount of kilojoules as their original product, it seems that we have created a society that believes low-fat food is equal to eating nothing.

As health professionals, it's sad to think that we have got the low-fat message across so poorly. Yes, fat has the highest kilojoules per gram of all nutrients, so it would seem reasonable that eating less fat would reduce kilojoules and therefore weight, but only if there isn't any added protein or carbohydrate to the product and we eat the same size serve. A common misbelief is that because it's low-fat or diet, you can eat more. I'm sure you have heard the theory that 'it's low-fat so I can eat twice as much'. If we're trying to control weight and prevent lifestyle diseases, this concept doesn't work too well.

The low-fat concept has been grabbed by food companies with two hands. Although a food may be low-fat, it still contains similar kilojoules to the original product. It's always important to check the nutrition information panel on the label to see whether the sugar or protein content have been increased. When checking similar products see how closely the kilojoule contents compare. If they are close, it will be smarter for your health to choose the original product.

Health halo and fat

We don't believe in feeling guilty about eating unhealthy foods; however, we do believe that proactive eating is important. Think about how many times you've been given something tasty where the offer was accompanied with 'it's low-fat'. A local café close to our office recommends its low-fat cheese every time we ask for none. We are sure this tempts many patrons to change their mind, but it still adds at least an extra 400 kilojoules. In one day, this isn't too much of a problem, but over the year it adds up.

When we notice that a food is low-fat or healthy, we tend to eat a much larger portion than we would normally. This has been said to be the reason that the French manage to maintain weight while eating fat to their heart's desire. They eat rich food — but in very small portions. In Western countries like Australia and the US, we know that when people think something is healthy they eat more of it. Researchers from the Cornell University Food and Brand Lab noted that when participants ate a 'healthy' choice from Subway, they actually ate more kilojoules overall than if they ate a normal, 'unhealthy' choice from McDonald's.

When you are about to eat something that is healthier, or you think is healthier, make sure you don't eat a larger portion, and don't get the extra additions that you'll surely be offered. Look at the kilojoule value rather than the fat value to decide the best option for you.

Fat and satiety

As well as eating more due to the health halo that comes along with foods that sport health and nutrition claims, low-fat foods are generally not as filling as full-fat options.

Fat slows the digestion of food and therefore processed low-fat products generally have a higher glycaemic index than full-fat products. This means that full-fat products make us feel full for longer, and deliver energy to our cells on a more consistent basis.

For some products, it's worth going lower fat than the original product to reduce some of the kilojoules, for example, having low-fat milk or low-fat cheese instead of the full-fat versions. In cooking, choosing low-fat options is also recommended. However, unless there is a medical need to go to a no-fat level, you may be making it more difficult to lose weight and maintain weight loss.

Our recommendation is to go for the middle of the road — the low-fat options, but not the 'no-fat' options. If you have a low-fat treat like muffins or chocolate bars or ice-cream, they still count as if they are a treat food — not an everyday option.

Fat and satisfaction

When you plan to eat a treat food and you want the 'real' version, the truth is that you may not be psychologically or emotionally satisfied, even if you're feeling happy. This can end up with you eating more or eating a variety of 'light' options, resulting in more being consumed overall or still having your original craving.

If you have your treats planned proactively, you will be able to prevent reactively eating the tempting low-fat treat foods that show up in your life. Our suggestion is to plan the treats that you really love. Aim to stick to one treat a week eaten away from the home, and one free meal. This will keep you satisfied with your lifestyle-eating plan and allow your weight loss to be sustainable and, above all, good enough.

Fat proteins and added fat

Fat protein foods that are naturally high in fat, like meats, chicken skin and dairy products, add unnecessary kilojoules to your diet. We need you to trim the fat from meats, remove the skin from chicken and choose low-fat dairy options. Fat protein foods can be replaced with lean protein foods for better weight loss results, but will not affect your hunger because protein is also satiating.

Added fat from cooking with lots of oil, butter, ghee or cream is also not helpful for weight loss. Because fat is high in kilojoules it's not worth serving with your meal for additional flavour. A simple rule is to not eat fat on fat. This means not having high-fat foods with other high-fat foods. For example, don't eat butter or margarine with peanut butter; cream and ice-cream; mayonnaise on butter or margarine; creamy sauces on fatty meats; or cheese with a non-lean meat.

Benefits of fat in weight loss

Fat in foods is often the evil stepsister. For years, we have tried to reduce all fat from our diets. However, the type of fat in food is much more important than the amount of fat in a food. Some fats even have health benefits, so we don't want to reduce all fat from our diets.

'Good' fats

Good fats can help to reduce cholesterol and heart disease, improve mood and depression, and manage inflammatory diseases such as arthritis, irritable bowel syndrome and diabetes. Eating good fats also adds to the flexibility of our skin and can reduce the signs of ageing. Good fats include omega-3, polyunsaturated fats and monounsaturated fats.

'Bad' fats

Bad fats contribute to heart disease, obesity, liver diseases and inflammatory disorders. Bad fats include saturated fats and trans fats.

Increasing 'good' fats

When you aim to increase your intake of healthy fats, you will naturally reduce your intake of unhealthy fats, and this is good news for your body and health. The easiest way to do this is to replace bad fats with good fats. If you add good fats to your diet without reducing bad fats, you may actually increase the kilojoules you eat.

Fats as medicine

Omega-3 fats have been shown to have therapeutic benefits in conditions like heart disease, arthritis, depression, diabetes and attention deficit disorders. The amount of omega-3 required to have therapeutic benefits varies depending on your condition, and it's best to seek advice from a health professional about this. However, most people without a medical condition can have up to 1 gram of omega-3 (three standard fish oil capsules) per day for health benefits.

Fat in the Good Enough Diet

For the reasons we have just explained, we don't want you to cut out all the fat from your diet. In fact, we want you to eat good fats by replacing bad fats. We all need some fat in our diet, but this doesn't mean you need to add a lot of fat. By the time you use some oil in cooking and eat whole foods that are naturally high in fat, such as nuts and avocado, you will have enough fat in your diet. Moderate fat is good enough to lose weight in the Good Enough Diet. Table 6.1 lists some examples of good and bad fats.

Table 6.1: good and bad fats

Omega-3 fats (Good)	Mono-unsaturated fats (Good)	Poly-unsaturated fats (Good)	Saturated fats (Bad)	Trans fats (Bad)
• Fish • Seafood • Linseed (flaxseed) • Walnuts • Pecans • Hazelnuts	• Avocado • Olive oil • Macadamia nuts • Game meats (e.g. kangaroo)	• Nuts • Seeds • Wholegrains • Canola	• Any fat solid at room temperature • Farm animal fat • Dairy fat • Butter • Chicken skin • Coconut oil • Palm oil • Ghee • Pastries • Biscuits	• Solidified 'good' fats • Deep-fried food • Highly processed foods

Takeaway tips

- Look at the number of kilojoules rather than fat content on nutritional labels.
- Ensure your portion size doesn't increase when you eat low-fat food.
- Don't be reactive to 'but it's low-fat' justifications about choosing low-fat foods.
- Look at more than the kilojoule content when choosing a product. Consider how filling a food is, whether it contains fibre and whether you will eat more because it is not what you really want.
- Don't add fat that is not needed.
- Don't eat fat on fat.
- Cut fat from meats and remove skin from chicken.
- Replace bad fats with good fats.
- Use avocado as a spread rather than butter.

The Good Enough Diet

- Use hummus as a spread rather than butter.
- Replace some farm meats with game meats.
- Eat fish three times per week.
- Eat nuts as a snack or add to cereals for breakfast.
- Use healthy oils such as olive oil, canola oil or sunflower oil for cooking.
- Grill your food or stir-fry in small amounts of oil rather than baking.

Chapter 7

THINK BEFORE YOU DRINK

When we want to lose weight, we often take more notice of our exercise and food but neglect the kilojoules that sneak into our diet from extras, particularly extras from things that don't fill us up — such as drinks. It's amazing how many kilojoules can be packed into a glass of liquid. Reducing the kilojoules from drinks can be very effective for great weight loss results.

Silent sabotage

Lara Kristenson knows this all too well. She works as a sales representative for a big pharmaceutical company, requiring a number of meetings with doctors, nurses and pharmacists daily. She came to see us six months before her wedding because even though she was pumping iron in the gym and pounding the pavement, her weight was just not shifting. Obviously something was wrong with her diet, but Lara just couldn't work out what. Her meals were healthy — cereal for

Silent sabotage (cont'd)

breakfast; salad or a sandwich for lunch; and a lean meat, vegetable and wholegrain carbohydrate meal for dinner. Unless she was attending a work function, which was once or twice a week, she cooked meals for her fiancé and herself at home.

At university she had managed to maintain a svelte 63 kilogram body, despite an unhealthy diet. Now, she was eating better than ever and exercising constantly, but couldn't budge from 75 kilograms. She was trying hard. Desserts were cut out, and she said no to the cakes, muffins and biscuits that were offered at sales meetings.

When we looked at Lara's diet we could immediately see why her weight wasn't shifting. Combined with the glass of juice, three—*yes, three*—lattes throughout the day and a glass of wine at night, it didn't matter what she was eating, the kilojoules from her drinks covered half of her daily kilojoule allowance to lose weight.

Using conservative glass and cup measurements, Lara was drinking almost 3000 kilojoules per day. We needed her to eat about 5500 kilojoules in total to drop the weight she wanted to for her wedding. If Lara was drinking large milky coffees, like many of us do, her kilojoule damage could have been much worse. To put this into context, 3000 kilojoules is like eating an additional three medium-sized chocolate bars per day.

To burn this off Lara would have to walk an extra 10.5 kilometres per day. So, we made a couple of changes. Lara didn't mind swapping to long blacks or peppermint tea for meetings with clients. She drank water with squeezed lemon juice for breakfast but drew a line on her special 125 millilitres glass of wine at night and stuck to this daily. She drank soda water from a wine glass if she felt like anything extra. By doing this we cut out 2700 kilojoules per day. Only small changes to her food and exercise regimen were needed to get to a 4000 kilojoule deficit, and her weight loss started as we expected.

> Lara couldn't believe it was that simple. Because her food and exercise hadn't changed dramatically, she didn't find that she was hungry. Occasionally she would have her favourite lattes; however, she limited them to when she was having coffee with her fiancé or friends rather than during work.

Liquid energy

Most of us are aware that there is plenty of sugar in soft drinks and cordials, and we tend to limit these in our diet. As health professionals, we find that these don't cause the biggest problems in weight management. Not because they are unhealthy, or high in sugar — they are, but most people will drink these in moderation because they realise they're high in sugar. In saying that, while a 375 millilitre can of soft drink containing 675 kilojoules was once the norm, 600 millilitre bottles outsell these and contain over 1000 kilojoules. See appendix B for the kilojoule content of these types of drinks, including varieties of milk.

Coffee fix

Like Lara, many Australians meet people for coffee and the variety of coffees is starting to resemble a wine list in complexity and variations. While instant coffee with a dash of milk was once the norm, we're now drinking lattes, cappuccinos, double shots and extra talls, with every variety of milk imaginable.

It's difficult to give up coffee completely and some research shows that there are health benefits; in particular, two cups of coffee per day can assist with diabetes prevention. However, with the quantity of kilojoule-containing milk and added sugar in its regular and/or syrup form, caffeine is the least of our worries.

The trouble is that coffee is seen as a drink — just like water. But it isn't water, and doesn't contain the kilojoules of water. Because many coffees have the kilojoules of treat foods, they should be classed as such. Once we add some sugar, get a muffin or slice to accompany our coffee, we are in for double the kilojoule trouble. See appendix B for the kilojoule content for a full range of coffee drinks.

Alcohol

So now that we have completely ruined your humble relaxing coffee break, let's see if we can do that to your Friday afternoon drinks as well. We all know that drinking too much alcohol isn't good for us and is linked to diseases such as high blood pressure, stroke, heart disease, liver disease, diabetes, depression, kidney disease, malnutrition and cancers — just to name a few! However, there is good news for those of you who don't mind the odd beverage or two. A little bit of alcohol may increase the length of your life and improve your health. The benefit seems to be largely related to the social aspects of drinking, stress relief and the anti-blood-clotting properties of alcohol, and not merely due to the antioxidants, such as those in red wine that was originally hypothesised.

So when does drinking turn from healthful to harmful?

Although everybody's ability to process alcohol is different, reductions in heart disease and stress-related illness have been seen in men who drink between two and four standard drinks per day. For women (due to not only their smaller size, smaller liver but also a lowered ability to break down alcohol) these benefits are maximised with one to two standard drinks per day. Everyone should allow for at least two alcohol-free days per week, and just because you refrain from drinking during the week, it doesn't mean that you can indulge in a big weekend and still reap the rewards! Our bodies and our liver can only process a certain number of drinks at any one time — the remainder will cause harm to our body.

Alcohol and weight management

So, what's with the beer gut — and why are we starting to see this Aussie male characteristic affect so many women? It's not just the sugar like many believe. Alcohol contains nearly as many kilojoules per gram as fat (29 kilojoules per gram versus 36 kilojoules per gram). So if you pour your drink stronger, it's like asking for extra cream or butter. If we don't burn up these extra kilojoules, we will gain weight and store this extra energy as fat. See appendix B for the kilojoule content of alcoholic drinks.

But juice is healthy, right?

When questioning the amount of juice drunk by some of our clients, it is often defended with 'But juice is healthy, right?' and then after a little thought, 'I know it has lots of sugar in it...but it's natural sugar!'

It's an interesting comment, considering that sugar, including table sugar, comes from sugar cane. Yes, sugar doesn't take the same form as it is grown, but neither does juice when compared with fruit.

Why not juice?

Fruit juice is often advertised as having the goodness of four oranges in every glass—sadly, more often than not a lot of the goodness is left behind in the juicer and what we get is a load of sugar. Fruit juice contains the same amount or more sugar than soft drink and, yes, even if freshly juiced! Fruit contains a high amount of fibre, nutrients that are only useful if eaten in whole fruit. All of this goodness is left in the juicer to be discarded instead of eating whole fruit that can prevent and manage many illnesses.

A small glass of juice should be the most that both adults and kids drink daily. Juice really becomes a problem when it replaces water as our main drink.

What about juice bars?

Fruit contains around 300 kilojoules per fist-size piece, so it's a great snack as it has lots of benefits and only contributes to 3 per cent of the kilojoules we need daily. However, a regular-size juice from a juice bar contains 1700 kilojoules to 2200 kilojoules. Wow!—in one regular juice that's more than two chocolate bars worth of kilojoules. That's not a drink, that's a meal in a cup! See appendix B for the kilojoule content of a full range of juices.

How much fluid do you need?

Although health professionals recommend that you drink a couple of litres of water daily, the amount required is very individual. It's important to drink before you get thirsty, as once you are thirsty you're already starting to get dehydrated, which can mean lower energy, poorer concentration and headaches. The other common myth is that tea and coffee are dehydrating. This isn't true. In a cup of coffee or tea, remove the effect of the caffeine, and there is still at least 150 millilitres of positive fluid.

To ensure you're drinking enough, your pee should be clear, not bright or dark yellow. For most people, this takes about two litres per day (including tea and coffee), but will change depending on how active you are and the temperature where you live.

What about diet drinks?

Diet cordials and diet soft drinks are okay occasionally; however, drinking diet soft drinks may increase your preference and intake for sweet foods. Caffeine also increases cortisol, a stress hormone that promotes weight being distributed to your middle region.

Caffeine-free diet soft drinks are an option when you're drinking at home. If your choice of drink when eating out or meeting friends is alcohol, juice or 'real' soft drink, diet soft drink is your best option. Again, getting used to the taste is just about familiarity. Both Coke and Pepsi have new sugar-free options that taste closer to the 'real' drink.

What about tea?

Herbal teas have additional health benefits. For example, green tea is packed with antioxidants, peppermint tea can help with stomach issues and chamomile tea can help with relaxation. Tea has the added benefit of being very low in kilojoules; however, don't be fooled by iced teas and fruit fusions, which have added sugar. You can make your own iced teas instead to get the benefits of flavour with lower kilojoules.

Drinks and the Good Enough Diet

We suggest you include warm drinks like black coffee (with a small amount of milk) or tea when you feel like some comfort. Drink a glass of water when you have the opportunity and when you feel hungry. Have a glass in the morning and half an hour before meals. When you go out, drink a diet soft drink or soda with lemon or lime.

Takeaway tips

- Many drinks should actually be classified as foods, not drinks.
- If you're drinking any kilojoule-containing beverage, always choose a small size.
- Choose non-kilojoule-containing drinks as much as possible.
- Don't keep kilojoule-containing drinks in the house or at work.
- If you must have a sweet, fizzy drink, choose diet varieties of soft drinks.
- Choose low-fat or skim milk in your milky coffees.
- Don't forget to count the kilojoule-laden drinks as snacks (or meals).
- Choose low-kilojoule alcoholic drinks if you are drinking alcohol.

Part II GOOD ENOUGH EXERCISE

Chapter 8

Productive exercise

Health professionals rarely use absolutes, such as 'you must eat this many kilojoules' or 'you must exercise at this exact time of day'. However, an absolute that we strongly believe is that you can no longer see exercise as dead time. In our fast-paced world we no longer have the luxury of simply exercising for exercise sake. We need to use exercise to kill two birds with one stone. Time is gold to us. We need to marry exercise to other parts of our life, whether it is social, family or business time. This mindset is key to being good enough.

To practically embed this in your life follow this four-step process:

- *Step 1.* Look at the different parts of your life. Everyone has their own unique list; however, here are some you may relate to:
    - family
    - work
    - study/education
    - interests/hobbies

- social life
- relaxation
- spiritual/personal.

📌 *Step 2.* Decide which part of your life you are going to marry with exercise so you're covering two parts at one time.

📌 *Step 3.* Ensure that it is practical and doable.

📌 *Step 4.* Get into it!

Following are some case studies that successfully combine business with exercise.

Taking the boardroom to the beach: CEO breakfast

Jordan Hawke is the executive general manager of Asteron, a proactive and innovative insurance company. Jordan's hectic work and travel schedule constantly gets in the way of his ability to exercise. To overcome this he has many different strategies to combine exercise with other parts of his life. On Wednesdays he meets with one of his senior managers for breakfast in Manly. They meet at 6.30 am for a surf and then a run. Then they grab breakfast and talk about the business and what they're going to focus on the following week. Jordan finds that after this exercise they feel much more creative and innovative. He says, 'I am surprised about how many great ideas we come up with over breakfast. I'm sure it's a combination of the exercise, fresh air and feeling good!' In addition Jordan also believes that spending this time with his senior manager cements their relationship and how they work together.

The gift that keeps on giving

Adam is often asked by up-and-coming speakers to meet with them for advice on how they can begin professional speaking. This causes him

> a lot of tension as it takes up so much time. However, he was offered a lot of advice when he started, so likes to give back to other people. To overcome his frustration, when people call him he no longer meets them for coffee, and instead they accompany him when he walks his dog, Tilly. The outcome is that people get their advice, Adam doesn't lose any business time and Tilly has another person to love.

Walks and talks

> One of Tara's mentors is Mia Sadler, a very successful businesswoman and dietitian. She has been one of Tara's mentors for the last five years. Whenever they get together for a mentoring session or to catch up, they do a 'walk and talk', meaning their two-hour meeting is spent walking. The great thing about this arrangement is that neither woman loses time in her already busy schedule, they share ideas and solve problems, they chat about life in general, while both get their exercise for the day.

In these case studies none of the work meetings involves sitting down for coffee and cake. Often when we meet people we feel compelled to consume high-kilojoule beverages, which makes it incredibly hard to lose weight. The great thing about active meetings is that not only are you burning lots of energy, you're also taking in fewer kilojoules.

Take your brain to the gym

Many people have to juggle full-time work with study, which can be a huge drain on your time and most likely will take up the time that you would normally spend being active. However, exercise and learning is a match made in heaven.

When you exercise there is a huge influx of blood and nutrients delivered to the brain, altering its biochemistry so your brain is ready to learn. In particular, exercise increases a chemical in our brain called brain-derived neurotrophic factor (BDNF), which is essential for learning and memory. So every time we exercise, 'miracle grow' is sprinkled on our brain to help it learn (the University of Copenhagen recently also showed that the presence of BDNF helps us to reduce our body fat levels). A number of schools in the US have discovered this and are now getting their students to do high-intensity exercise first thing in the morning before class. Interestingly, the children do best in the subjects that immediately follow these exercise sessions. So by combining exercise and study, you can not only control your body fat levels but also maximise your learning.

We were recently in a gym where a girl was on an exercise bike while reading a textbook and using ear plugs. When she finished we asked her what she was doing. She told us that she was doing a post-graduate degree in medicine and that if she didn't study at the gym, she would never make it there. The downside was the loud music in the gym as it made it hard to focus. To fix this she wore ear plugs and found that she got completely lost in the material she was reading and would go over time on the bike because she became so fixated on her study. She then went on to say that she retained much more information during her gym study than any other time that she spent studying.

Welcome to the digital age

The development of the iPod has significantly changed our lives. One of the best things about it is that we can listen to audio while we exercise.

And with the rise of the internet, you can find a podcast on almost anything, from how to do home taxidermy (we are not making this up) to understanding how to produce wine. You can pick up university lectures you have missed or that are held on the other side of the world. You can learn a language; even listen to your favourite radio show. There is a world of education out there that you can access while you are exercising. Exercise will never be dead time again.

The balancing act

A friend of ours, Nick, is an executive with two young children who decided to do an MBA (as if he didn't have enough on his plate). After he began he realised that he had very little time to do all of the required reading. He tried to do it late at night but this prevented him from spending any time with his wife. And exercise was a thing of the past with his jam-packed life.

Nick started to record his lectures on his iPod so he could listen to them on his commute to and from work. Unfortunately, due to the recording quality, he found it very hard to listen to the lectures on the bus. He then decided to walk to work, which took him about 45 minutes and was quicker than if he took the bus (his bus commute was 55 minutes in traffic, plus waiting time and time to get to the bus stop). He also walked through the back streets, which were quiet so he could hear his lectures. In addition he downloaded podcasts that related to the topics he was studying. For example, he listened to podcasts from Harvard University on emotional intelligence. He found that this method not only helped him get back into exercise, it also helped him salvage some family time.

The mobile book worm

At the start of 2005 Tara set herself a goal to read a book a week. She was a year into her dietetic business and had been told by business mentors that this was the way to get the information needed to achieve her goals in life. With her multifaceted life she found it difficult to physically sit down and read a book. Her solution was to download the book to her iPod and listen to it. She then went one step further and combined the audiobook with exercise. She only listened to the audiobook when she was exercising. The average audiobook is around seven hours in length, so if she has listened to a book a week she knew that she had completed at least seven hours of exercise in that week. Both Tara and Adam are training to swim the English Channel in 2012 and have already put in an order for waterproof iPod shuffles. The trouble now is not the time to read, or retaining the information, but having enough audiobooks available for Tara to listen to. This has been great because she has both stretched her genre consumption and learnt information that she would otherwise not have had time for.

Social time is a team sport

Some friends of ours had recently had their second child and noticed that they rarely saw other friends who were in a similar family situation. They had become social recluses and, as you do, they had put on some body fat since they had been married. In an effort to kill two birds with one stone, they got their friends together and set up a netball team for a midweek competition, with one person from the group taking a turn to mind the kids while the game was being played. A result the group has noticed is that everyone has started to lift their activity level outside of the games so they are in better shape to play. When we asked them what benefit they got out of setting up the netball team, one member replied, 'I don't even notice I'm exercising because we are having so much fun and we're so focused on the game. From a social front we are so much closer as a group. I not only feel healthier but my happiness and wellbeing are far greater from the social interaction'.

Moving meditation

A client of ours, Christine Archer, is one of the most vibrant women on the planet. To say she lights up a room is an understatement. She is incredibly energetic and goes at a million miles an hour. One thing she has always struggled with is her inability to relax and find down time. She has tried meditation and relaxation classes; however, she struggles to sit still and relax. She actually finds this extremely stressful. However, what she has found is that she feels incredibly relaxed and calm after having a swim. The rhythmic movement of the swimming motion combined with the silence underwater is incredibly relaxing. Christine uses her exercise time as her relaxation time. She certainly kills two birds with one stone.

Escape the world for some personal time

Sue is a senior executive with three young children and a husband who works full time. As with all working mothers, personal time is a rarity. Early Sunday morning is the only time that Sue has a moment to herself. She gets up at 6 am and goes for a walk. She says that being up while everyone else is asleep and the golden sunshine at that time of day make her feel like a million dollars. During this time she thinks about her world and what is going on. She says that it's almost her spiritual time, where she checks in with herself and recalibrates where she is at and what she's focusing on. The family gets a sleep, she feels great and everyone wins.

Takeaway tips

- Make a list of the different areas of your life that you want to give more time to.
- Determine a strategy to combine that part of your life and exercise.
- Ensure that you have the right tools to make it work. This may mean buying an iPod, downloading podcasts to iTunes or organising exercise times with a friend.
- Get busy.

Chapter 9

YOUR EXERCISE PROFILE

Whether we know it or not we all have a relationship with exercise. Some people love it, some tolerate it and some would rather stick bike spokes in their eyes than do it. You know that exercise is good for you and you 'should' do it. Yet, it can be hard to introduce into your life.

Your relationship with exercise hinges on two main factors:

1. *Your introduction to exercise.* If you were the 'fat kid' or the 'uncoordinated kid' at school, you probably felt bad about being involved in sports and exercise. You have negative memories and negative emotions attached to being active. But if you were the school jock, you will have fond memories of exercise and it can be a source of pride and positive emotions.

2. *Your self-image.* Humans have a basic need for our behaviour to match our self-image or identity. In other words, you need and want to act like the type of person you think you are or want to be. Some people come into our clinics and say, 'I am just not an exercise-type person'. If you have this view, you are less likely to stick to a regular exercise program.

So while it is important to know what type of exercise will help you lose weight, it's worth spending a moment to understand your relationship with exercise. In our exercise clinics, we have found that people generally fit into six different exercise personalities, which describe their relationship with exercise.

Exercise-free zone

If you are in the exercise-free zone category, you believe exercise is as much fun as doing your taxes. In fact, exercise is not a word in your language. You never think about it or talk about it, and neither do many of your friends or family. Winston Churchill describes this well: 'Every time I get the desire to exercise, I lie down and it goes away'.

Is this you?

- You do no formal exercise at all.
- You refer to yourself as 'not an exercise-type person'.
- You don't own a pair of sports shoes or any exercise equipment.
- You say things about exercise like 'exercise doesn't work', or 'it's not worth the effort'.
- The thought of exercising rarely enters your head.
- You would choose not to go somewhere if it meant walking to get there.
- You might drive home from the shops if you couldn't park near the entrance.
- You will get a taxi or bus to your destination, even if it's close.

If you answered yes to three or more of these entries, this is your exercise personality. To change your approach it's important to consider why you have developed this attitude, and how might it be holding you back from improving your health. Start by challenging your thinking and beliefs — are they rational and realistic?

To change your approach follow these action steps:

- Make it enjoyable. Choose an activity that is going to be fun for you or change it so that it will appeal to you, like exercising with friends, learning to dance or getting involved in physical volunteer work such as the State Emergency Services.

- Take it easy. Don't try to do too much. If you overdo it, you can have a further negative experience and reinforce your unenthusiastic attitude towards exercise.

If you *don't* change your approach:

- You won't make any significant improvements towards your relationship with exercise, which is okay if exercise genuinely doesn't appeal to you.
- You may still lose weight if you stick to your diet, but your low fitness will still increase your chance of heart disease and other illnesses.

Yeah, but …

If you're a 'yeah, but' exerciser, you would love to get out and exercise but… You set goals to exercise, and even set the alarm to get up, but something always stops you. You would have exercised this morning, but your excuse is…

- 'I've had a hard week, I need a rest.'
- 'I've been good for two days. I deserve a sleep in.'
- 'Is that rain I can hear?'

Is this you?

- You often take your exercise gear to work but never use it because life always gets in the way.
- You find yourself saying 'I'll start tomorrow', 'I'd exercise but I don't have time', or 'It's not a good week for me'.
- You feel out of control in your life, and your life runs you rather than you running your life.
- You contribute to the gym charity fund, where you have a membership and pay fees monthly, but never actually exercise there.
- Your personal trainer sacked you for cancelling too many appointments.
- You aim to exercise five days a week and only make it to one or two sessions.
- You own a treadmill but it serves as an unusually shaped clothes rack.

If you answered yes to three or more of these entries, this is your exercise personality. To change your approach you should focus on actually achieving manageable exercise goals and building habits that will get you there.

To change your approach follow these action steps:

- Make a list of your most common excuses and assess how valid they are.
- Write a list of strategies to overcome these excuses.
- Realise that the plan doesn't have to be perfect, just take some regular action.
- Reconsider your goals. Maybe they are unrealistic and you're setting yourself up to fail. Reduce your expectations a little — just focus on getting a regular pattern happening, even if it means exercising once a week — which would be a 100 per cent increase on the week before!
- Find a type of exercise that is more appealing and you are more likely to do it.
- Start exercising with a friend or exercise physiologist to hold you accountable.
- Consider how you spend your time during the day — maybe there are things you can change to make sure you do have time for exercise.

If you *don't* change your approach:

- You'll keep jumping from plan to plan and never commit to any of them.
- You'll continue to set unrealistic goals and you'll keep getting little result.
- One day, you'll decide it's all too hard and will stop trying.

Hard slog

If you're a hard slog exerciser, you are exercising regularly and achieving all of your goals, but enjoyment is not high on your list. In fact, you wonder how people can say they actually enjoy exercise. Each exercise session involves a lot of blood, sweat and tears, and you have to psych yourself up before heading out the door. When you go for jog, smiling, relaxed people who merely glow without sweating pass you. You want to inflict grievous bodily harm on them — if you could only catch them!

Is this you?

- Before you exercise you have a feeling of dread.
- You often say to yourself 'does this ever get easy?', 'When will I start to enjoy it?' and 'I can't seem to get into a groove with exercise'.
- During exercise you are uncomfortable and sore.
- The only reason you exercise is due to your Olympian-like willpower.
- You have to focus strongly on the weight loss benefits to keep going.
- You don't see exercise as a source of enjoyment.
- Your exercise doesn't vary from week to week.
- You usually exercise alone.

If you answered yes to three or more of these entries, this is your exercise personality. It's great that you have the willpower to exercise, and that you value the weight loss and health benefits from exercise. However, you can make exercise a much better experience if you change your strategy.

To change your approach follow these action steps:

- Realise that you may be doing too much, too soon, and overwhelming your body with exercise before it can adapt and catch up. Review your exercise program and remember that building up gradually is better.
- Check that your exercise suits your body and even your personality. For example, muscular, stocky, solid people rarely suit long-distance running and can be better at more powerful activities, such as resistance training or sports that require agility; while tall, lean people rarely suit power-based exercise and can be better at endurance sports like running, rowing, swimming or dancing.

- Some people prefer social sports, such as golf or tennis, while others have a preference for individual activities like jogging and/or swimming. Know what your preference is and do something that brings you joy or makes you laugh. You will get better results when you do the exercise that suits you best. Try different forms of exercises or even different sports to inject some fun and to work out what you like best, so you do enjoy it!

If you *don't* change your approach:

- You will always see exercise as something you do not and will not enjoy.
- You may sustain an injury from too much or the wrong type of exercise.
- Your willpower may slump and you'll stop entirely.
- You will become the Darth Vader of the exercise universe where you turn to the dark side and try to turn as many people against exercise as you can!

Exercise evangelist

If you are an exercise evangelist, you're the Richard Simmons of the exercise world. Remember him? No — try googling him! He lost a truckload of weight by changing his lifestyle and proceeded to tell the world about it via his TV show. He was like the Energiser bunny on overdrive, in tiny shorts, as he ranted and raved about the wonders of exercise. You may not be quite as over the top, but you do think exercise is a gift from the heavens. You have a regular exercise habit and you enjoy and look forward to your regular exercise bouts. You are seeing great results and life is great.

Is this you?

- You look forward to your exercise sessions.
- When you miss a session, you get grumpy.
- You get an exercise 'high' after the session.
- You schedule in your exercise sessions and consider them a priority.
- Your friends are regular exercisers.
- You incorporate exercise into social activities, such as walks or tennis with friends.

- You say things like 'I love training', 'I'd never miss a session', 'I feel so much better after doing it' and 'I'm an exercise-type person'.

If you answered yes to three or more of these entries, this is your exercise personality. Keep doing what you are doing! But if you haven't reached your weight loss goal, it's time to alter your routine to get further results and avoid stagnation and boredom. You may benefit from trying a new activity or simply increasing the intensity of the exercise you're doing now. Or, you might need to focus more on your food and ensure you are fuelling your exercise correctly.

If you *don't* change your approach:

- You could get into an exercise rut, where you do the same thing over and over and don't add variety or progression into your program.
- It could affect the continued benefits you have received from your exercise and therefore your results. Variety is the key.

Yesterday's hero

If you are a yesterday's hero exerciser, you probably know who you are. Let's face it — we all know a *yesterday's hero*. You used to be fit and you used to exercise all the time, but you're out of the habit and haven't been able to get it back.

Is this you?

- You used to be fit, but not anymore.
- You have tried to get back into old habits but you can't manage it consistently.
- You often say to yourself: 'I'm just not that person any more', 'My lifestyle is different now — it's no longer suited to exercise', 'I just can't get back into my old routine' and 'I don't want to get involved, because I'm not as good as I used to be'.
- You look in the mirror and wonder who that overweight person is.
- You believe that you will never be as fit again.
- You believe that your change in circumstance or age is the sole reason you don't exercise any more.

To change your approach follow these action steps:

- Acknowledge that your life has changed and you need to find a new approach to get back into exercise. Stop thinking it's just a matter of doing what you used to do, or that you have to be as competitive/good as you used to be.
- Think about what you are able to change and what you can commit to. Remember what it was about exercise that you enjoyed and think about how you can get that again. For example, get satisfaction from the team atmosphere of a Masters Sport, group personal training or a semi-competitive organised sport environment.
- Consider having any injuries or even just creaky knees or shoulders looked at before you start exercise to avoid making those injuries worse.
- Don't start off with what you 'used to do' when training.

If you *don't* change your approach:

- You'll stay stuck in the past instead of moving into a new phase of your life.
- You'll miss out on recapturing the enjoyment you used to get from exercise.

Never again

If you are a never again exerciser, you don't exercise because you've had a bad experience in the past, maybe because of bad advice, bad trainers, not knowing what to expect or just overdoing it. Maybe you remember being extremely sore, or trying so hard but achieving very little. Whatever the reasons, at some stage you have said, 'Never again!'

Is this you?

- You had an injury due to exercise.
- You worry about stirring up the injury if you exercise.
- You believe that if you start exercising it is only a matter of time before you hurt yourself again.
- You think that exercise professionals are careless and incompetent and don't listen to you.

- You say things like 'All trainers are bossy and aggressive' or 'Exercise damages your body'.
- You think that any injury stops you from all exercise.
- You think that all exercise makes you really sore afterwards.

If you answered yes to three or more of these entries, this is your exercise personality.

To change your approach follow these action steps:

- Before you go any further, get your injury properly diagnosed and treated. We recommend seeing an exercise physiologist, physiotherapist or osteopath. Go to the relevant professional association's websites, as they usually provide a register of professionals in your area or who specialise in your injury.
- Find an exercise physiologist and talk to them about an exercise program that will work around your injury, not make it worse, as well as suit your body and your life. Their in-depth knowledge is what you need to get on the right path to exercise.

If you *don't* change your approach:

- Your injury will continue to trouble you.
- You'll never get to experience the benefits of a properly designed exercise program.
- You will find it hard to lose weight without exercise.

As you can see, everyone is different and their strategies to success are different. The first stage in changing your behaviour is awareness, and being aware of your relationship will help you identify what is preventing your weight loss.

When you know your exercise personality and accept the suggestions to make exercise more effective for you, you will be better able to keep to the program, ensuring your weight loss is sustainable.

Takeaway tips

- Understand your exercise personality.
- Do exercise that matches your exercise personality.
- Just because something worked for someone else, it might not be the right thing for you. In saying that, there is no harm in trying.

Chapter 10

THE BEST EXERCISE

We spend most of our day in negotiation mode. 'Do I take the stairs or the elevator?' 'Should I exercise now, or later?' 'Do I walk, jog or run?' 'Do I walk to my meeting or take a cab?' 'Yeah that's a great idea, but I have been good all week so I deserve a break.' We are constantly negotiating with ourselves about what behaviours we can get away with. It's kind of like we are both the parent and child — in one person. Now who wins most of the time with you?

For most people, the child often wins. This is because our default negotiation position is to try to get maximum benefit with minimal effort. We want to do the least amount of exercise we can get away with and we want to eat the most amount of tasty food we can. Our day even starts with a negotiation. Our performance research has shown that the majority of people wake up and instantly shift into negotiation mode.

The alarm clock goes off at 6.00 am, you roll over, press snooze and go back to sleep. It goes off again, you roll over, press snooze and go back to sleep. It goes off a third time, you roll over, press snooze, but instead of going back to sleep you shift into 'mathematician mode'. This is where you lie there and actually calculate in your head the latest time you absolutely must get out of bed. You lie there and say to yourself,

'I had a shower the day before last, that will cut out 15 minutes, brush my teeth, nah, I have gum in my drawer that will save another three minutes' and you come to the conclusion that in order to leave the house at 7.00 am you can get up at 6.55 am.

Because people gravitate towards negotiation, a common question we often hear is 'What is the least amount of exercise I can do and still lose weight?' This is a loaded question. Weight loss through exercise is all about how much energy you can burn in a session, a day, a week, a month, a year. The fastest way to lose weight is to exercise for as long as possible, at as a high intensity as possible. For example, 12 hours of gut-busting exercise will help you lose weight; however, few people are going to put their hand up for this one, and a little thing called *work* will get in the way.

Studies show that exercise is an essential component of fat loss — with the more exercise you do, the more fat you lose. Exercise seems to have a magic impact on fat loss! Let us explain. Weight loss comes from a deficit in kilojoules, that is, from burning more kilojoules than you eat. And people lose more weight when this deficit comes from exercise rather than just reducing the food you eat.

A group of researchers from Tasmania reviewed the relationship between exercise and weight loss. They found that you can lose weight via diet alone. However, when you combine diet and exercise you get better and faster results. To back this up we have seen the same thing in our clinics.

The following points are the current recommended exercise guidelines (4–5 days a week):

- 30 minutes of moderate exercise (brisk walking) to maintain health
- 45 minutes of moderate exercise to stop putting on body fat
- 60 minutes of moderate exercise to lose weight.

These guidelines are lower if we do vigorous exercise, like running. Instead you need to complete the following amount of exercise most days of the week:

- 20 minutes for good health
- 30 minutes to stop putting on body fat
- 45 minutes to lose weight.

The big question is are these guidelines accurate for you? Unfortunately, the answer is 'it depends'. Exercise helps us to lose weight, but how much depends on four things:

- how hard you exercise
- how long you exercise for
- your metabolic rate — how much energy your body burns
- how much you eat.

Recently we attended a conference, where an ex-Olympian was the guest speaker. He was discussing how to improve health, and although he had some good points, he was more of a de-motivational speaker than a motivational speaker. He was expecting everyone to be perfect, and everyone to have the willpower, prioritisation and time to exercise of an athlete. His first piece of advice was, 'If you can't exercise for an hour a day, you should forget about it — it's not worth doing at all'. He is wrong! These types of messages are not only stupid but dangerous. This attitude certainly goes against our good enough philosophy. Audience members who couldn't do 60 minutes of exercise per day just switched off, thinking that if they can't do an hour, why bother at all. They lost their motivation to exercise because they couldn't do an hour a day.

But if *you* can't do an hour of exercise per day, you should bother, because small amounts can make big differences, and after a while of building your time up, you'll be able to manage an hour a day.

The truth is that any amount of exercise will benefit your health and help with weight loss. Apart from burning body fat, exercise increases your energy levels and dramatically improves your mood. Some studies have shown that exercise can be more effective in the treatment of mood disorders like stress and depression than anti-depressant medication. If you do suffer from depression, we're not suggesting that you stop taking your medication, but you should start to exercise, as it will improve your mood. (You should always talk to your GP or psychiatrist before changing or stopping any of your medication.) Exercise can help you feel more energetic and optimistic, making sticking to any weight loss plan easier.

If you want to maximise how much body fat you lose through exercise, think of the following rules to be good enough.

Principle 1: must combine it with diet

All the research tells us that the best way to lose weight is to combine exercise with a kilojoule-controlled diet. However where we run into trouble is that food today is very dense in kilojoules, so it's easy to undo all the good work you do with your exercise. Having a large sports drink after exercise can negate the kilojoules burned during that session. Another pitfall is exercising well all week and deciding that you deserve 'a blow out' and eating a huge kilojoule meal to celebrate.

It is rare to have enough time to exercise as much as we would like with our busy lifestyles, so it's impossible to think we can eat anything we want and still stay slim. Some athletes we've worked with in the past can eat a huge amount of food without putting on fat. However, they do four hours of training a day. Other athletes can't lose weight, even if they are doing four hours of exercise per day.

When you try to lose weight just by dieting you will, without question, lose muscle mass and bone density. This is detrimental to your health and enhances the negative effects of ageing. Without exercise, losing weight will also reduce your ability to lose weight again in the future because as your active tissue (muscle) reduces, your metabolic rate also drops, making it harder for your body to adjust if you put weight back on again after losing weight. Exercising while you are dieting will reduce this loss of muscle and bone density and in many cases can also actually increase them or at least their percentage ratio. Exercise and dieting must go hand in hand.

Principle 2: the longer the better

The longer your exercise sessions are, the better. Why? Because you burn more kilojoules and the more kilojoules you burn, the more fat you lose. But let's give you some parameters to work with.

If you are exercising at a moderate pace, a study from Italy suggests that there is an exercise–weight loss tipping point beyond 30 minutes. This study involved 179 women (they all had similar metabolisms, age and health status) and looked at how different amounts of exercise affected their ability to lose body fat. One of the key things they did was control their diets so they were consuming similar amounts of food. The group of women who were doing around 30 minutes of exercise per day lost a tiny amount of weight and had only a moderate decrease in their waist measurement, while having great health improvements.

With this in mind, you could expect that if you did 45 minutes of exercise per day, you would lose at least the equivalent weight and waist measurements. Was this so? No! The group that did 45 minutes of exercise per day, lost twice as much body weight and more than three times the amount of centimetres from around their waist. Wow.

So the real message here is that a 50 per cent increase in the time you spend exercising will give you a 200 per cent or more increase in benefits. Any financial planner will tell you to get on board with this investment!

If you want to get exact, the women that had the most significant decrease in weight were walking at 6.4 kilometres per hour for 45 minutes. For most people, 6.4 kilometres per hour is a brisk walking pace. If you want to exercise at a moderate pace and maximise the amount of fat you can lose, this is your starting point.

If you can't fit in the 45 minutes and only have time for 30 minutes, we often get our clients to try to get in some extra exercise on the weekends. Going for long walks or hikes and making weekends active is a great strategy for both weight loss and enjoying your environment.

These examples will optimise your weight loss; however, if you can't do 30 minutes of exercise, 20 minutes is still going to give you some benefit. For example, if you planned to exercise for 45 minutes at lunch and your meeting goes over, leaving you only 20 minutes for exercise, still go for it! It is 20 minutes of energy you are burning. This is what the good enough philosophy is all about. Read on to discover some tricks that will allow you to decrease the amount of exercise you do but still get the same benefits.

Principle 3: the harder the better

If you really want to drop the amount of time you have for exercise, the solution is to increase the intensity at which you exercise. Go as hard as you can, huffing, puffing and sweating for the time you have available. An example is going for a 20-minute jog. However, if the thought of pounding it out for 20 minutes makes you nauseous, there is an alternative — interval training!

Interval training is when you vary the intensity of how hard you exercise. So you exercise at your normal intensity and then exercise much harder for a shorter period, then go back to your normal pace. For example, you walk at a brisk pace for three minutes and then jog for one minute (an interval), then go back to your normal walking pace.

There are no hard and fast rules on how you structure your intervals, and you can do any variation in your intervals. Table 10.1 shows some examples.

Table 10.1: interval training examples

Timing of intervals	Intensity 1–10 (1 = really easy, 10 = maximum effort)
4 minutes	5 out of 10
1 minute	8 out of 10
4 minutes	5 out of 10
1 minute	8 out of 10
Repeat for the rest of the workout.	

As your fitness level improves you can progress to the examples in table 10.2.

Table 10.2: further interval training

Timing of intervals	Intensity 1–10 (1 = really easy, 10 = maximum effort)
3 minutes	6 out of 10
2 minutes	8 out of 10
3 minutes	6 out of 10
2 minutes	8 out of 10
Repeat for the rest of the workout.	

You can add intervals to any form of cardiovascular exercise. For example, when cycling, cycle at a comfortable pace for 45 seconds and then go as fast as you can for 15 seconds, then repeat.

Why do we want to do it? Say you are walking for 30 minutes and you add intervals where you walk for four minutes at your normal pace and then jog for one minute. If you repeat this pattern for the full 30 minutes, by the end you will have completed six minutes of jogging.

Now if most people tried to do six minutes of jogging, they would be exhausted by three to four minutes and have to stop. However, because you have introduced it in short little bursts you still stay fresh but get the same benefit. As you get fitter you can start to lengthen the time of your fast intervals and start to reduce the time of your slower intervals. Also, no matter how fit you are, you can do this because you can make it relative to your fitness level.

A client of ours, Cherie, aged 86, was able to walk on the treadmill at 1.6 kilometres an hour. Have you seen a treadmill move at 1.6 kilometres per hour? It's barely budging! Every three minutes Cherie began including thirty-second intervals at 2.5 kilometres an hour. After six months of slowly increasing the pace of the intervals, she is now walking at 5 kilometres an hour for 15 minutes. Not bad, eh! Interval training allows you to work harder and greatly increase your fitness level, with the result that you lose body fat faster.

Here is some proof. A study conducted at the University of New South Wales showed the benefits of interval training. They took a group of young women and split them into two further groups. One group did normal exercise, the other group did interval training. The *normal* exercise group had to complete 40 minutes of cycling three times per week. The *interval* training group also cycled three times per week, but they only did 20 minutes and included some intervals. The intervals they chose were very short and close together. They did eight seconds of sprinting immediately followed by 12 seconds of pedalling as slowly as possible, repeated for 20 minutes.

This study continued for 15 weeks. At the end of the period they found that the *normal* exercise group doing 40 minutes of moderate exercise lost on average half a kilogram. In comparison the women in the *interval* training group that did half that amount of exercise but exercised in intervals lost 2.5 kilograms of weight. So if you are time poor, intervals are the way to lose weight.

Principle 4: pick the right type

Often when we think about exercise in relation to weight loss we think of activities like walking, going for a run or riding a bike. These are all forms of aerobic exercise (often referred to as cardiovascular exercise); however, exercise comes in many different forms. The other main form of exercise is resistance training, sometimes referred to as weight training. This is where your muscles have to contract hard to lift an object (bench pressing a weight) or to move your body away from something (a push-up on the floor or getting out of your chair).

While resistance training will give you amazing health results, such as strengthen your bones, prevent chronic disease, improve mood, keep your muscles functional, and increase heart condition, it is rarely prescribed by health professionals/trainers for people to lose weight.

Let's look at how resistance training stacks up in comparison to aerobic training in terms of weight loss. However, before we go any further, it's important to realise that every person responds to exercise and different types of exercise in a unique way. We have found a number of studies that reveal a large variation in the amount of weight loss that some people achieve within the same exercise program. Therefore, we need to realise that different types of exercise work for different people.

New evidence shows that when we do resistance training we use up a lot of energy and much of that energy comes from body fat. The other great thing about resistance training is that it uses up a lot of the glucose that is stored in our muscles. Why is this important? When your muscles are depleted of glucose, the next time you eat, the glucose you ingest goes to refuelling your muscles rather than being stored as fat. However, the benefits don't stop there. Following resistance training you can get an increase in how many kilojoules you burn while you are at rest and while you are asleep. A study in the US involved a group of people who completed an 11-minute workout of resistance training. They performed nine exercises (one for each of the major muscle groups — chest, legs, back and so on) in the 11-minute period. For 24 hours after the workout there was a significant increase in how much energy they were burning while at rest and while they were asleep. Hands up if you would like to burn more fat while you are asleep after just 11 minutes of exercise?

The challenge with resistance training is that most people who exercise in gyms follow the traditional body-building model. This type of training is designed to increase the size of your muscles. For example, you complete an exercise set, say 10 repetitions of bicep curls, you have a large rest (two to three minutes) and then repeat the exercise again. The rest is used to allow the muscle to recover from the previous set so you get the most out of it. Often you see people in the gym standing around talking (or looking in the mirror) in between sets. While they may be in the gym for an hour, they are actually only exercising for around 12 to 15 minutes. If your goal is weight loss and not building big muscles, this type of training is unacceptable. Your rest to exercise ratio is far too high.

When it comes to resistance training and weight loss there are three rules:

1. *Keep the rest in between exercises to an absolute minimum.* You are not trying to build big muscles, you are trying to lose weight. Because of this you don't need the muscle to completely recover before you exercise it again.

2. *Vary the muscle groups that you exercise.* Rather than do three exercises that work your legs, do an exercise for your chest, briefly catch your breath and then do an exercise for your legs, pause briefly, and then go straight to an exercise for your back, your shoulders and then your arms. Do resistance training in more of a circuit style, rather than in the body-building model where you do an exercise for your chest, rest three minutes and repeat.

3. *Train to failure.* This means that by the time you get to a certain number of repetitions you can no longer lift the weight. For example, if you're doing 15 reps on the bench press, choose a weight that by the time you get to the 15th rep you can no longer do any more. In terms of stimulating weight loss we've found that the 12 to 20 reps range is the best to stay in. The reason why you want to train hard like this is that high-intensity resistance training burns more energy and is thought to stimulate more of that post-exercise increase in energy burnt.

We have found the most practical way to use resistance for weight loss is to combine it with aerobic training. Following is an example of a gym workout that you can do to combine resistance training and aerobic training.

Start with 15 minutes on the bike doing intervals. Cycle at a normal pace for two minutes followed by one minute as fast as you can and repeat for 15 minutes. Then do one set of the following exercises with no more than 10 seconds' rest in between:

- bench press for 15 reps
- leg press for 20 reps
- back rows for 15 reps

- shoulder press for 15 reps
- squats for 15 reps
- upright rows for 15 reps
- leg curls for 20 reps
- bicep curls for 12 reps
- bench dips (just using your body weight) for as many reps as you can do
- jump on the treadmill and do 15 minutes with intervals
- after this repeat the entire resistance training circuit.

You can play around with this routine as much as you want. For instance, you could do 10 minutes of cardio work followed by the resistance training circuit, then repeat this circuit twice. If you prefer to do all of your cardio in one block, then do 30 minutes of cardio and then two circuits of resistance training.

This type of circuit can be incorporated in your outdoor training. If you are going for a walk or a jog, when you get to a park bench you can do a set of pushups on the bench, then go straight into a set of lunges using the bench for balance, and finally a set of bench dips. You can do this as many times as you like during your run.

Aim to incorporate resistance training into your aerobic training. Not only will it make your workouts more interesting, but it will also give your weight loss a boost.

In the last 15 years the popularity of yoga and Pilates has exploded. While yoga and Pilates are great for your health, body and stress levels, they are not the most effective ways to help you drop lots of body fat. I know that countless celebrities say the reason for their slim figures is due to these exercise techniques; however, the reality is that these exercise forms just don't burn enough energy compared with aerobic or resistance training. We're probably offending yoga and Pilates enthusiasts, who are likely to argue that they work just as hard, but these exercise forms will never burn as much energy as high-intensity aerobic or resistance training.

Takeaway tips

- Exercise is essential for weight loss.
- Any amount of exercise will help you in your effort to lose weight.
- Exercise improves your mood and will help you to stick to your weight loss plan.
- Exercise must be combined with diet to maximise your weight loss.
- The longer you can exercise the better your chance of losing weight.
- Exercise as hard as you can to increase how much weight you lose.
- Add interval training to your exercise routine.
- Focus on aerobic training and resistance training when you design your exercise routine

Chapter 11

ANYTIME IS THE RIGHT TIME

You probably wonder when the best time to exercise is. We are often asked when you should exercise for maximum weight loss. Our response is always the same — 'whenever you can exercise is the best time'. Sometimes in our desire to be perfect we miss out on doing what is good enough.

Scientific studies have shown that if you exercise in the morning in a fasted state (not eating since the night before), you will burn more body fat than if you exercise after you have eaten. The theory is that when you are fasted your insulin levels and your blood glucose levels are lower. These two factors put the body in a state where it relies more on fat as an energy source. This is great, but although this has been shown in a laboratory, in the real world there may be no actual difference.

Some people exercise perfectly on an empty stomach, so this may be the right option for you. Other people find that they can't exercise at as high an intensity when they haven't eaten, therefore they actually burn fewer kilojoules because they can't invest as much energy than they would if they were exercising at a time when they felt more comfortable.

In reality the difference may be as small as a slight increase in kilojoules of fat burnt. You need to weigh up the benefits for yourself. If exercising on an empty stomach first thing in the morning is not a problem for you, go for it. However, many people find it very difficult to exercise at this time, and can't exercise for as long or as hard. Try not to over analyse it. Anytime is the right time to exercise. Choose a time that suits you best — your body will thank you for it.

Incidental exercise

Incidental exercise is a form of exercise that we just fit into our day. It is simply looking for opportunities to move and taking those opportunities. Many websites say that incidental exercise makes a big difference to how much weight you lose. When we googled the question 'Does incidental exercise lead to weight loss?', plenty of websites confirmed yes, but we could find no studies in any scientific journals that backed this up.

One observation we made was that each website that confirmed the positive offered the same list of suggestions for increasing our incidental exercise. They commonly were:

- get off your bus two stops before work and walk/run the extra distance
- get up and go talk to a colleague at work rather than call or send them an email
- take the stairs rather than the escalator or elevator
- park your car at the furthest part of the car park and walk to the shops
- get rid of your remote control and stand up every time you want to change channels
- leave your car at home and walk to the shops

The good news about incidental exercise

A new research project conducted by Baker IDI Heart and Diabetes Institute, the Cancer Prevention Research Centre at The University of Queensland and Medibank Private showed that the average office worker spends 77 per cent of their work day in a seated position.

Add to this the fact that most Australians travel to work in a seated position (train, bus and car), and outside of work are also seated the majority of the time (TV and computer viewing). In other words, we are sedentary for most of our day. The problem is that when we are sedentary our metabolism is pretty much turned off, our muscles aren't doing anything and we are burning only a small number of kilojoules. Researchers are saying that this lack of movement increases a person's chance of chronic diseases (diabetes, heart disease, hypertension), as well as orthopedic issues (neck, shoulder and back problems). In particular, TV viewing time is related to your risk of heart attack.

Incidental exercise is proposed as the solution — simply be more active in your day. There are definitely health benefits to incidental exercise. For example, some studies have shown that even standing rather than sitting may improve our body's ability to process cholesterol. And with the huge rates of orthopedic issues in this country, regularly standing up and moving around will lessen your chances of an injury in the workplace.

Our verdict is that in terms of your health and physical wellbeing, incidental exercise is a great idea and you should do it as much as possible.

The bad news about incidental exercise!

Most of the ideas in the list of suggestions for increasing our incidental exercise are very inconvenient. The good enough philosophy is all about doing things that work with our lifestyle rather than disrupt it, so pursuing this list flies in the face of that philosophy.

Get off your bus two stops before work and walk/run the extra distance

Most of the businesspeople that we work with are simply always in a rush. If getting off the bus two or three stops early adds 10 minutes to their already rushed commute, they are not going to do it. Also if you are working in a professional capacity and it is summer, you are going to sweat, or if it's raining, you'll get wet, and this will affect your appearance, not to mention add even more time to getting yourself composed once you reach the office.

The Good Enough Diet

Get up and go talk to a colleague at work rather than call or send them an email

This is a huge interruption for you and your colleague. The average person is interrupted every three minutes, so if you contribute to this, you're not going to be popular. You may be able to do this a couple of times a day, but if you did this every time you needed to contact people, you would get nothing done.

Take the stairs rather than the escalator or elevator

A good suggestion, but impossible if you are travelling with luggage. The challenge with this one is that the average person is presented with this choice only a couple of times a day. Worth taking on but the impact is not that high. Plus climbing anything over five floors will get you a bit hot and bothered.

Park your car at the furthest part of the car park and walk to the shops

Good to do if you are on your own and you don't have to get a lot of stuff. Walking through a car park with kids can be diabolical; also if you get a dodgy trolley it can be a real slog.

Get rid of your remote control and stand up every time you want to change channels

Next! Really, has anyone in the history of the world ever done this? Most people with new flatscreens wouldn't even know where the buttons on their TV are located.

Leave your car at home and walk to the shops.

A great idea if you don't have to carry a lot of shopping. This really hampers your ability to buy a lot of groceries.

Back to the bad news!

The second bit of bad news is that when it comes to weight loss, the impact of incidental exercise is quite small.

Let's consider the kilojoules burnt climbing the stairs as opposed to riding the escalator. If climbing the stairs takes 15 seconds, by the end you would have burnt around 4 kilojoules (this calculation is for a 70-kilogram person). Therefore, if you choose to take the stairs and not the elevator on four occasions, you will use around 16 kilojoules of energy. A piece of bread contains around 335 kilojoules, so unless you are going up and down the stairs about 30 times a day the impact on your weight loss is next to nothing.

A new movement is encouraging people to spend more time standing, even going as far as encouraging people to use desks that you can adjust the height of so you can type while you stand. Other suggestions include standing up when someone comes to talk to you, or standing while you use the phone. Once again, the health benefits would be great, but they're not going to allow you to drop much body fat.

The difference between sitting for an hour and standing for an hour is around 145 kilojoules. This amount of energy is equal to less than half a slice of bread. If you stood for an entire eight-hour day (which very few people can do), not sitting down at all, a 70-kilogram person will burn an extra 1170 kilojoules. That's three slices of bread. If you could do this all day every day, it will make a significant difference to your ability to lose weight. However, what is the chance of this happening? Most people complain when they have to stand on a train for 30 minutes. We recommend standing up throughout the day when you are on the phone or when people come to speak with you at your desk. Just bear in mind that this does not give you licence to pig out at the end of the day.

A problem with incidental exercise is that we develop a 'health halo' around it. We think 'I've been on my feet all day so I can have lots of dessert tonight' or 'I don't need to walk, because I was up and down the stairs all day'. Why do you think you see overweight labourers who do hard physical labour all day? Because they overcompensate by eating too much food! Meat pies for breakfast, three sandwiches for lunch, and all washed down by a truckload of soft drink.

The official verdict is that incidental exercise is great for your health on the whole. If you have the choice to do it and it's convenient, always choose movement above not moving. However, realise that you are not going to lose a lot of weight from it. The key philosophy of the Good Enough Diet is to do things that will give you maximum results with minimal disruption to your life. With this in mind, if your focus is weight loss, incidental exercise for the average person is not going to get you great results and may be a constant interruption throughout your day.

What's the solution?

Factor longer periods of activity into your day. Also be more productive during the day, which may mean less incidental exercise but will allow you to take the time to go for a walk at lunch or get home half an hour early so you can go for a quick jog.

Even exercising during the day is a great idea. Halfway through the day our brain starts to get tired, simply because we were not designed to sit still and use our brains without movement. Studies have shown that people who exercise halfway through the day return to work more focused, more refreshed and more creative. Some studies in particular place the improvement in productivity at 15 per cent.

Too busy to do this? Let's look at two examples that show how busy people fit in movement during their day.

The team that exercises together bonds together

Adam, co-author of this book, was doing a project with IBM when he discovered that the Health and Safety Team got together daily for a walk at lunchtime. During this time the group would talk business and discuss the challenges they were facing. Not only did the group lose body fat but they also felt better when they returned to the office. Some ran, some power walked and some ambled. But they were all out there. There was also a cultural benefit, as doing something together each day as a team brought them closer.

Dr Fiona Wood

Dr Fiona Wood is a high-profile burns surgeon from Perth. She came to local fame and was awarded the Australian of the Year in response to her efforts with the Bali bombings burn victims.

To say that Dr Wood is busy is an understatement. As well as being the director of the Western Australian Burns Service at Royal Perth and Princess Margaret hospitals, she is also Chair of the McComb

Foundation and heads the research team at the Burn Injury Research Unit at the University of Western Australia. She mentors other upcoming surgeons and lectures to university and corporate groups throughout the world. Oh, we forgot one thing—at the time of our interview, Dr Fiona Wood had six children, all living at home!

With a lifestyle like this you would think exercise is the last thing on her mind. However, the most amazing thing about Fiona is that on most days she exercises for around an hour and a half. Her exercise of choice is early morning cycling.

When you look at Fiona's life it's hard to comprehend how she can fit all of this into her day and still prioritise 90 minutes for exercise daily. We were curious about this and asked her about it. 'Fiona, with so much going on in your life how can you afford to exercise for an hour and a half?' She replied, 'That is the wrong question. A better question is with all this going on in my life how can I *not* afford to exercise for an hour and a half each day. If I get up and ride my bike the day is better. I can remember times in my life when I couldn't exercise. I didn't have as much energy, I couldn't get through the day as well and I wasn't as effective. Also I noticed that my mood was lower and I was less tolerant of my family and co-workers. My family know when I haven't been exercising. They say, you haven't been riding, you are grumpy. Being fit allows me to keep up with my hectic life'.

Fiona always exercises in the morning, because it helps her to feel good about herself. At 7.30 am, she can look back and be proud of how much she has accomplished already.

Fiona's attitude towards keeping herself fit is exciting. One day she was in a board meeting. On this day the directors had a 90-minute lunch break. Because Fiona carries her exercise gear with her everywhere, she was able to eat her lunch in half an hour and put on her joggers and get in almost an hour of walking. While her colleagues sat around and chatted, she got an hour of exercise, some fresh air, sunshine and a clear head.

Dr Fiona Wood (cont'd)

Fiona also had this attitude when her children were younger. When her kids were doing swimming training, she would go off to the gym, or jump in the pool in one of the spare lanes. On surf club Sundays, Fiona would run with her kids while they were warming up.

Fiona just couldn't see the point in sitting around doing nothing while waiting for her children to finish sport. She thought that she may as well get some exercise in too — and she did. Surprisingly, some parents would see what she was doing and join in with her.

Like many women, Fiona initially felt selfish about taking time for herself to exercise. So when her children were young, she exercised with them. One thing they often did was 'Park Crawls'. She would have one child in the backpack, two in the pram and the rest on little bikes. They would set off from the house until they reached a park. They unpacked all their gear, ran around and played games, packed up and headed to the next park where they did the same thing. They would do a huge circuit of parks until they came home worn out. She just participated in everything they wanted to do — rollerblading, bike riding and surfing.

Australia has such a great climate that it's easy to be active with your kids. Fiona used to walk everywhere with them, too. The great thing out of all of this is that her children are now really active and also play lots of sport.

A great time to inject exercise is around the 3 pm energy slump. One of the factors that affects our energy levels is the amount of glucose that we have in our blood. The reason for this is that our brain exists on glucose and nothing else. Our brain makes up about 2 per cent of our body weight but consumes more than 20 per cent of the glucose that we eat.

We see a huge drop in our glucose levels during midafternoon. How often do you get tired at 3 pm? When our glucose levels are low, we feel tired, can't focus and generally our productivity stinks. At this time it's a great idea to get up and move, it will make you feel better and reignite your energy levels.

There are three keys to making this work:

1. *Bring your exercise gear to the office!* Always keep extra gear at work.
2. *Have somewhere convenient to change.* Most companies have showers and change rooms, but if not, exercise at a level that doesn't cause you to sweat too heavily. If you do get sweaty and a shower isn't an option, towel off in a toilet cubical and apply deodorant liberally.
3. *Get over the guilt.* Often when we take a break at work we feel guilty about it. We fear that people will think we are slack. Don't worry, legal publishers LexiNexis released a report in 2010 that showed that the average full-time employee only worked productively for two and a half days per week. So while you are out exercising, your co-workers are probably just staring at their screensaver or watching YouTube.

Exercise boosts productivity and culture

Adam, co-author of this book, walked into the foyer of Announcer, a friendly financial planning business, and was greeted by the receptionist, 'Can I help you?' 'Yes, Adam Fraser here to see Andrew Rocks.' 'Certainly, please take a seat while I go get him.' After a brief period of time an employee walked past and noticed that Adam was sitting alone. He asked, 'Are you being taken care of?' 'Yes I am just waiting for Andrew.' 'Great, is there anything I can get you in the meantime?' 'No I am fine.'

Shortly after another employee strode past. 'Hi, is someone looking after you?' 'Absolutely, just waiting for a meeting.' 'Brilliant, if you need anything just ask.'

This did not happened twice, it happened four times in the short period of time that Adam was waiting for their CEO. The bizarre thing was that these people were planners, not the support staff. In all of the foyers Adam had waited in, this had never happened. The place seemed to have a buzz to it. When Andrew came out Adam was amazed by his

> *Exercise boosts productivity and culture (cont'd)*
>
> energy. As they sat down, Adam told him about what had happened in the foyer, and he didn't seem the least bit surprised. He said, 'Yes, we're very proud of our culture'. Adam asked why everyone was so energetic. He replied, 'We really focus on them being active in their day. On Monday morning we all do a boot camp session together to shake off Mondayitis. Also each day we encourage them to get out and exercise between 2 pm and 4 pm, when they are paid to be active. Wednesday and Friday we play basketball or touch football as a team. The other days they are encouraged to go to the gym or get outside for a walk. We found that their productivity and energy levels started to slip. But if they go outside and exercise, they come back more energised, happier and more productive. Not only does this keep them healthy it also makes them more effective and gives our culture a massive boost'.
>
> We cannot be productive at work for the entire day — it's impossible. But why not give your productivity a boost and lose some body fat at the same time?

Takeaway tips

- The best time to exercise is the best time for you.
- Incidental exercise is great for your health but not for major weight loss.
- Don't replace planned exercise with incidental exercise.
- Be on the lookout for gaps in your life that present themselves and try to fill them with activity.
- Involve the kids and the whole family.
- Move as often as you can and the longer the activity you do, the better.

Chapter 12

Have fun with it

Think for a moment. Why do we have emotions? What is the point of them? Many people say they make us human, but it goes deeper than that. We have emotions for many reasons, some of which are:

- they allow us to communicate
- they make sense of situations
- they give us signals
- they allow us to bond with people
- they allow us to care.

However, the most significant thing they do is drive our behaviour and control our motivation.

Emotions drive our behaviour

At a very basic level the primary function of an emotion is to help us survive. Emotions can hijack the brain and cause us to react and overreact very quickly. For example, if we are walking through some long grass and we see a snake near our feet, the emotion of fear will take over our thought processes and cause us to move very, very quickly. So, in effect, the emotions we feel throughout the day control and drive our behaviour.

Let us prove it to you. Have you ever bought something you didn't really need? Of course you have! Think back to when you stood in front of it, logic started to kick in … You don't need it. You can't afford it. It's not practical. You have something just like it … Yet, you walk out with it. Why? Because of the emotional kickback you get from making the purchase!

Logic makes us think, but emotion makes us buy. We buy products, we join social networks and we follow a certain trend because of the emotional satisfaction we get from doing those things.

What is branding? It's the emotional attachment you have to a company and how you emotionally relate to it. This is why some women pay $1000 for a pair of Manolo Blahnik shoes or $5000 for a Dolce & Gabbana handbag. They don't logically think, wow, that's a great price for a bag! They are compelled to buy because of how it will make them feel to have that bag or wear those shoes.

An executive from Harley-Davidson once said, 'The company doesn't sell motorcycles. What we sell is the ability for a 43-year-old accountant to dress in black leather, ride through small towns and have people be afraid of him'.

Why do men buy a Harley? Because of how it makes them feel! If you were buying a motorcycle and you used logic, you would buy a Japanese motorcycle (cheaper, more reliable and runs forever), but instead you buy a Harley because of how it feels to buy, ride and own a 'Harley'.

Why do people eat certain foods? Because of how it makes them feel to eat those foods. Why do we sit on the lounge and eat chocolate after a break-up? Or drink alcohol after a hard day at work? Because of the emotions we feel when we do those behaviours.

Your ability to stick to any health plan or diet is all about the emotions you attach to that new behaviour. Every decision we make each day goes through a logic versus emotion arm wrestle. While on a diet, if we pick up a doughnut, the logic part of our brain says, 'Put that down, it will make you fat, this is not part of your health plan'. Then the emotional part of the brain kicks in. It can go one of two ways. It will back up the logical part: 'Don't even think about eating that. You have bought a new dress for Sally's wedding, you will feel terrible if you can't fit into it'. Or it can go against the logic: 'One won't hurt. Doughnuts are my favourite. I feel so good after I eat a doughnut that the world always seems better'.

If your emotions want you to have the doughnut, logic will be powerless to stop you and the logical part of your brain will have to sit by and watch as you inhale the doughnut.

The key to changing any behaviour is to regulate the emotions you feel when you are faced with a decision. The emotional payback from sticking to your new behaviour has to be greater than the emotion you will feel when you break it.

Emotions control our motivation

Our desire to stick to any lifestyle change is controlled by the emotion we relate to that task. Have you ever set your alarm to get up early and exercise, yet stayed in bed?

What emotion do you feel when the alarm goes off? Most likely apathy, sadness, anguish, disgust and irritation. So — you stay in bed! Then you feel guilt! But the logical part of your brain comes to the rescue and justifies why you should stay in bed: 'I'm having a hard week', 'I deserve a lie in' or 'Is that rain I can hear?'

'Actually tomorrow would be better for me, yes, yes, tomorrow I will definitely get up tomorrow.' Compare this scenario with the day you fly to Italy for a holiday and you have to be at the airport at 5.30 am. How easy is it to get out of bed that day? You wake up every hour on the hour thinking, 'Is it time to go yet? Should we get there four hours earlier just to be safe?'

What is the difference? The emotions you have attached to your overseas holiday are elation, happiness, excitement and enthusiasm. The emotions you attach to getting out of bed to exercise are the complete opposite.

The problem with trying to be perfect and going on extreme diets is that you're creating a terribly boring and unenjoyable experience. You can only do this for so long until the emotional part of your brain demands some attention — by getting revenge from taking you to a pizza joint for a blow out. This is the beauty of the good enough approach, as it stops you from feeling those huge emotional swings.

Unless you attach some sort of positive emotion to your activity, you won't be as motivated to stick to it. The following case studies describe this perfectly.

Become a team player

Keith Taylor loves weight training. He could lift weights all day. The challenge with Keith is that he is a little slack with his diet (he loves alcohol and isn't willing to compromise). This is fine because he lifts weights four times a week and therefore his weight is stable and he's quite healthy. However, he is carrying about 5 kilograms more than he would like. In the past the only thing that would help him drop weight is doing cardio exercise three times a week.

This is where we run into trouble. Firstly, Keith has old football injuries that make running impossible and walking not much fun. He also detests doing any form of indoor cardio training—the bike, cross trainer and step machine are all out. We finally discovered that he really enjoys swimming. Keith trekked off to the local pool to pump out some laps. He enjoyed being in the water but after 10 minutes he became very bored and wanted to get out (nothing with Keith ever went easy). In a last ditch effort we signed him up for a swim squad, a group that gets together three mornings a week and swims with a coach. Keith loved it, loved it. He liked the social interaction and never got bored because the coach kept changing the program so they never did the same thing. He even stuck to it through winter, swimming in an outdoor pool. 'Last month I found myself waking up at 5.30 am. It was 4 degrees celsius outside and very windy, making it even colder. I climbed out of my nice warm bed, drove to the pool, paid my entry fee, changed out of my warm tracksuit and Ugg boots and climbed into an outdoor pool to swim for 90 minutes. As I climbed into the pool a realisation hit me: What the *hell* am I doing! Why am I subjecting myself to this torture? I must be insane! The worst part is I do this three times per week.

'Then I realised I am not insane—it's because I belong to a team. Doing the squad is bigger than just exercise for me. I feel part of something. I like the other people in the squad, and they have become my friends. We organise get togethers outside of swimming, we compete in ocean swims over summer. The cold seems to even bring us closer as we bond over the fact that it is absolutely freezing. One thing I know for certain, there's not a snowball's chance in hell that I would do it if I were getting in that cold water all on my own. The emotional pleasure I get from doing the squad is what keeps me motivated and keeps me consistent.'

Emotional buy-in

Peta Harold had gained 20 kilograms since she left school. Being a working mother she always found it hard to fit in exercise and stick to any eating plan. Through Facebook she discovered that a group of old friends had organised a 10-year school reunion. She was very excited to catch up with them; however, she was worried about what people would think of her weight gain. With three months to go until the reunion Peta knuckled down to get fit and lose some body fat. Every time she didn't feel like exercising she would think about how good she would feel about herself at the reunion. She did the same when she felt the desire to break her diet. The emotional drive to look good at the reunion was greater than the emotional payback for staying in bed or eating a treat.

It may take time

Most people who continue to exercise on a regular basis get to the stage where the physical performance of exercise is the emotional driver. Physical activity is a mood enhancer. After we exercise we see a large spike in our mood and happiness. In fact, some studies have shown that physical activity is more effective than medication to treat depression. However, it takes a couple of weeks to get to this level.

When we start exercising we tend to go through three phases of how we feel about exercise:

1. *Discomfort phase.* This is when you do not enjoy the exercise while you are doing it and you feel sore and uncomfortable afterwards.

2   *Physical phase.* You still don't enjoy the exercise while you do it but afterwards you feel good.

3   *Psychological phase.* At last you feel good during the exercise and you feel great afterwards. If you have to miss an exercise session, you notice that you don't feel as good.

If we reach the psychological phase, we tend to exercise for life. The big challenge is that most people give up on exercise in the first or second phrases and their emotional relationship with exercise remains a negative one.

Consider the following tips to make your emotional relationship with exercise a positive one.

Have a clear goal to work towards

By giving yourself a challenge to work towards you will be more emotionally engaged. Whatever type of exercise you are performing, look for an organised event to participate or compete in that suits your fitness level, such as a fun run, an ocean swim or a walk for charity. You could even train for a holiday that involves physical activity. One of the best ways to see a country is by bike. Why not incorporate your holiday with a cycling trip? There are even some organised trips, many that require you to raise money for charity before going on your adventure. These trips can include hikes, running, cycling or serious trekking. Excellent fun to meet new people and help a great cause.

Join a group of like-minded people

When we share an experience with a group of people the emotional aspect is intensified. For example, comedies are funnier at the movies than watching them at home because there are more people around you laughing and enjoying them too. Sporting events are much more compelling when you are watching them live because your own emotions feed off the emotions of those around you. If you join a training group, you are far more likely to commit to train because of the camaraderie of the group. No matter where you live, there is bound to be a group you could join, whether it is a triathlon club, a running group, hiking group, line dancing group or a martial arts club.

Create your environment

One thing that can make you enjoy your exercise more is the setting in which you do it. Are you more likely to stick to your walking program if you walk around suburban streets or within a beautiful park? Always look to improve the environment in which you exercise. You may be more willing to exercise if you plan to exercise somewhere lovely. For example, why not escape peak-hour traffic and take a detour along the beach for an hour or so?

Get wired for sound

Gadgets like iPods have changed the way we exercise. While you are active you can listen to your favourite music, a podcast of your favourite radio show or some comedy. Your exercise time will fly by and dramatically increase the experience you have.

Make it social

Involving your friends or loved ones is always the best way to give your exercise attitude an emotional boost. In our fast-paced society it's so hard to find time to connect with friends and family. Why not combine the two?

Give back to others

There are a string of organisations that allow you to raise money for charities by competing in athletics events. Organisations like Can Too and Inspired Adventures create experiences out of marathon running, trekking or cycling. Getting involved in these events will not only get you active in training for the experience, but also allow you to meet others you can exercise with when you get home, and of course give you the opportunity to give back to the community or raise money for a good cause.

Takeaway tips

- Our emotions control our behaviour and our motivation.
- Whatever changes we are trying to make to our lifestyle must have strong and positive emotions attached to those reasons to ensure we stay motivated to make those changes.

- Ensure that the goals you want to achieve are very clear and specific.
- Feed off the emotions of other positive like-minded people who are trying to make the same changes as yourself.

Chapter 13

DRESS FOR SUCCESS

One of the challenges that overweight people face is that the exercise advice they receive is given to them by people who have never been overweight. If you are overweight it feels different to exercise than if you are thin. When you are overweight, your body moves differently. You are not as agile and you find it hard to do many things, but most of all parts of your body seem to have a mind of their own and when you stop moving, that doesn't mean every part of you stops moving. All this movement leads to chafing, blistering and rashes in places you can't talk about at the dinner table.

Trainers and health practitioners don't think about this — first of all because they have never experienced it, and second because they don't want to have the conversation. This chapter looks at how to make exercise comfortable.

When exercising there are three things that make exercise uncomfortable: hot conditions, cool conditions and friction.

Hot conditions

As summer rolls around and daylight saving kicks in we tend to be more active and spend far more time in the sun. While we welcome the hot days and sunny weather, they bring some significant dangers, such as skin damage and heat stress.

Exercising in hot conditions is vastly different from exercising in cool conditions. When we exercise the body generates heat that it needs to get rid of; add hot weather to the mix and you can get a lot of heat building up in the body. When you have more heat being absorbed into the body than is lost, you run the risk of heat stress.

The following explains how the body gets rid of heat:

- *Step 1.* When your temperature starts to rise, more blood is pumped towards your skin to try to cool your blood down. This is why your skin gets redder in the heat.

- *Step 2.* Once the blood gets near the skin it relies on the outside environment to take the heat away. Usually it is the air around our body that absorbs the heat. If we are in water it is the water that absorbs the heat.

- *Step 3.* If the surrounding air or water are not enough to cool us down, the sweat glands kick in. You have about four million sweat glands over the surface of the body. When sweat comes in contact with our skin, the hot air makes the sweat evaporate and we get a cooling effect. The amount of sweat that is evaporated from the skin depends on:

    - how much skin is exposed (the more skin you expose to the air the faster you cool down)

    - how humid the air is (when humidity is high, the air is saturated with water and the evaporation off your skin is reduced; a sign that sweat is not being evaporated is when you have beads of sweat rolling or dripping off you)

    - speed of the air over the body (the quicker the speed at which the air moves over our skin the quicker the heat is lost; this is why fans cool us down more than still air).

When you can't get rid of excess heat it starts to build up in your body and you are at risk of heat stress.

Dress for success

Here are some simple tips to follow in the summer months to protect against heat stress and skin damage.

- *Get your timing right.* Avoid exercising in the hottest part of the day, between 11.00 am and 3.00 pm. Early morning or late afternoon is the best time to get active in summer.

- *Wear the right gear.* Exposing lots of your skin to the environment helps to maximise evaporation; however, it leaves you at risk of sunburn. This problem has been solved by a number of companies that have produced an excellent range of exercise clothing that feature moisture wicking and breathable material to allow you to regulate your temperature better. Some clothes are also treated so that they have UV protection, equal to wearing SPF 15+ sunscreen. It is essential to have good-quality exercise clothing that will protect you from the sun's damaging rays while also keeping you cool. You will find them in any good sports store. Don't try to cover up in many layers of clothing. This will just make you hotter, preventing you from exercising.

- *Stay hydrated.* The most effective defence against heat stress is adequate hydration. Proper hydration levels help to maintain the right plasma volume in your blood to keep circulation and sweating at an optimal level. Before you head out to exercise it's a great idea to consume at least 500 millilitres of cold water. During exercise drink about 250 millilitres of water every 15 to 20 minutes. Take a water bottle with you if you are not sure if water will be readily available. You can also get bum bags that hold water bottles, and leave your hands free to swing for greater comfort. Sports drinks such as Gatorade have been shown to enhance rehydration particularly in hot and humid climates. Good sports drinks contain between 6 per cent and 8 per cent of carbohydrate and as high as possible in sodium (aim for above 20 millimoles per litre). Some sports drinks are glorified cordial with too much sugar and not enough salt. However, sports drinks do contain kilojoules, so if you are not exercising for a long time (less than two hours) or not at high intensity, you won't need anything more than water. If you need some flavouring, add some fresh mint, cucumber, lime or lemon juice to your water. However, if you are doing really intense or long sessions or long-day hikes in the heat, you may benefit from drinking a sports drink.

When exercising in warmer temperatures, foot care is important as there is a greater chance of your feet sweating. Sweaty feet are more susceptible to:

- increased friction between your feet and your shoe
- cracking and splitting of the skin, especially between the toes
- fungal infections like tinea, as these love warm, wet and dark areas.

In addition, another hurdle is that feet tend to swell in the heat, especially as the day goes on. This essentially means that in the summer months you are putting a larger foot in your shoes, which creates uncomfortable rubbing and friction and more chance of foot damage.

Here are some footwear tips for summer:

- *Stay dry.* Regularly change your socks so that they stay dry during exercise. Choose socks specifically designed for exercise, that draw moisture away from the feet. There are many brands, although Thorlo socks are great.
- *Wear higher socks.* Some socks are too short and can slip down into your shoes. This can create extra blisters.
- *Air out.* Make sure you air and dry out your shoes after exercising.
- *Allow for the swell.* When buying shoes in summer, buy them in the afternoon when your feet are at their most swollen.
- *Get the best.* The quality of your shoes is not something you should compromise on. Make sure your shoes fit well and are the right type for your feet. We understand the importance of aesthetics, but when it comes to sports shoes, this shouldn't be a deciding factor.

Cool conditions

One of the biggest challenges to a regular exercise routine is cold, miserable weather. We have all woken up early in the morning and strapped on our runners, only to hear that freezing cold wind — suddenly the excuse board comes out and we convince ourselves to stay in bed. Fortunately, we are very lucky that our skin is waterproof!

Because it's cold, and we wear more clothes, there can be the tendency to exercise less over the winter months. Following are some helpful tips that will motivate you to exercise even when it's freezing:

- *Dress right for the weather.* If you are keen to exercise outdoors rather than in the confines of a gym, you will get warm but those first few minutes can be hard to take! Dressing in layers means that you can remove them after you have started and you get warm. A polar fleece vest can help to keep your trunk warm but allow your arms to remain cool. Long-sleeved windproof jackets prevent wind chill and can be tied around your waist after you warm up.

- *In winter, aim for the middle of the day.* If you can start work earlier and move your exercise to the middle of the day, not only will you get a well-deserved break from work but you'll get to see the sun.

- *Do your exercise at home in the evenings.* You'll be out of the weather and can start and stop as you need to. Also you can save on your heating bill!

- *Don't forget to drink water!* Just because you don't feel as hot, or you may not be sweating (as much), doesn't mean you don't need to rehydrate yourself!

- *Be careful when exercising in the cold.* People with injuries or arthritis may find that the cold aggravates these conditions. Even people with otherwise healthy muscles and joints can find that their risk of injury increases when it's cold, so make sure you do a really good warm-up to prepare yourself before going for it. A warm-up should last for about five to 10 minutes, and consist of light-to-moderate activity, specific to the exercise/sport/activity you're about to do; for example, if you're about to run, start with walking and build the speed up gradually.

What if I get sick?

Avoiding the winter colds and flus can be harder than avoiding telemarketers! When to return to physical activity after you have been ill can be hard to gauge. If you get the dreaded flu or cold, resume your activity once you have fully recovered. Starting back too early may not give your body sufficient time to fight off those bugs. A good guide to judge when you are ready to return is when you have been able to do a few full days of work without feeling you've been hit by a truck or worse for wear the next day. Start with a light program or about 50 per cent the capacity of what you would normally do and if that's okay, return to daily activity. This can be hard to do but it's really important to get back into the habit of exercising regularly. Build from this light daily activity to the full intensity of your previous activity, rather than all at once, especially if it's been a few weeks since you were able to be active.

Friction

When you exercise, the rubbing and bobbing of body parts can be extremely frustrating. The less this happens, the more comfortable you will be. Even when exercising in 'perfect' conditions, you will find exercise easier and more effective if you can reduce friction. One common thing that our clients do is decide to wait until they've lost weight before they buy exercise gear, or wear baggy clothes to hide their bodies from the world. This is not the right approach.

If you are female, having a sports bra that fits well is of vital importance. If you have a large bust, wear a crop-top-style bra over a sports bra for added support. Support may also be required for men, and can be achieved by wearing a tight sports singlet. There are also specific sports tops for men that help support your body and keep the wobbly bits stable in areas more likely to need it when exercising. This can be worn as your top or underneath a breathable shirt.

If you are overweight, regardless of the intensity, you will sweat. Wear clothes that will help to keep you dry. There are many options that wick moisture away from the skin and are designed to keep you cool.

Now, these are probably the last thing you want to wear, but they will add hours to your exercising regimen — bike pants. Lycra bike pants will become your best friend. Even the legs of those in the healthy weight range rub together, and this creates chafing and bleeding. Many of our clients refused to wear them initially, but once they tried them, they never went back. You can wear them under shorts or pants, and they will stop the fabrics and/or your skin sandpapering your legs.

Compression garments are relatively new, but very popular among athletes. These provide additional benefits, particularly for those who have joint conditions, or take extra time to recover from exercise.

CW-X is one brand that creates compression tights that also give you the benefit of recovery. Tara has a joint condition, and after numerous knee reconstructions and arthroscopies found it difficult to run. Since these tights support her knees and calves, running is now one of her most enjoyable activities. You can buy compression garments that cover whole legs and whole arms, or anywhere in between.

Chafing creams, such as Neat 3B Action Cream, will come in handy when you start exercising. Often an afterthought following a rash or blister, chafing creams can be used in spots that may rub, such as between breasts, under your bust, between legs and on your bottom if cycling or horse riding. If you do get a rash or blister, make sure you keep them clean and dry, and cover them if you are doing any more exercise. This will save them from becoming infected, and really ruining your new-found love of exercise.

Takeaway tips

- Don't wait until you lose weight to buy appropriate clothing for exercise.
- Prioritise exercise clothing before you start your regimen.
- Have clothes appropriate for exercise in the heat.
- Have clothes appropriate for exercise in the cold, rain, snow or wind.
- Discuss the uncomfortable parts of exercise with your health professional, as they may have helpful options.
- Use chafing cream in spots that rub.
- Wear compression garments to reduce muscle fatigue and enhance recovery.

Part III GOOD ENOUGH MINDSET

Chapter 14

POSITIVE MINDSET

Due to the work that we both do, we have had the opportunity to work with some of the most talented and senior businesspeople in the country. These people range from professors and CEOs to multimillionaires. What many have in common is despite being ridiculously competent in other areas of their lives, when it comes to their health and losing body fat they do some incredibly stupid things. Not to be disrespectful but it's like aliens have come down, stolen their brains and removed their ability to have any logic or sophisticated thoughts whatsoever. They turn into morons that will believe anything and do the silliest things.

We have been mentoring John, a CEO of a large multinational company and responsible for thousands of staff. He is a genius who has turned the company around and achieved amazing results. Unfortunately, he has put on a large amount of weight in the last five years. We asked him to fill out a food diary. Upon analysis we noticed it was his large intake of alcohol that was the problem. When we asked him about this he said, 'Nah, it won't be the alcohol because I drink red wine not beer'. 'What do you mean?' we asked. 'Yeah, I don't drink beer because it's high in carbs, but red wine is low in carbs and good for me so that won't be making me fat.'

First of all, carbs are not the enemy, second, beer is not that high in carbs. Third, red wine still contains kilojoules (see chapter 7), and if you drink the amount that John was, of course he would put on weight. Absolutely red wine will make you fat if drunk in excess. We couldn't believe such a ridiculous statement would come out of the mouth of such an intelligent man.

A female executive was approximately 30 kilograms overweight. We sat down with her and worked out a great eating and activity program for her, that was not only achievable but at the same time very effective. She started the following Monday. On Wednesday she ran out of her blood pressure medication. Since she was too busy to go back to the doctor, she was no longer taking her medication. The type of medication she was taking was a diuretic, which basically reduces the amount of fluid in your body. By Friday her weight had shot up 4 kilograms (obviously due to no longer taking the medication). We explained the situation to her and why her weight went up. However, this did nothing to calm her hysterical reaction. She claimed, 'The program isn't working and we need to change it. If we don't, I am going to keep getting bigger and bigger. This is a disaster!' Clearly she wasn't looking at the situation logically. What was the result? She went back on her medication, the extra fluid was reduced in two days and she calmed down. This came from one of the most talented and brilliant businesswomen Australia has ever produced. She can handle a board of stuffy old men but when it comes to her health, her emotions take over and she loses logic.

A huge block to weight loss is that people interpret victories and setbacks incorrectly. The fallout is that they lose logic and their behaviour becomes erratic and ultimately sabotages any attempts to lose body fat.

Be consistent

The key to any weight loss strategy is to be consistent. As much as we hate to say it, if you stick to any of the ridiculous diets out there, you will lose weight. Why? Because all of them get you to eat less and move more. So whether it's the soup diet or the 'don't eat anything white diet', stick to it for long enough and you will see some results.

But how do you get consistency? Control the voices in your head! It's all about how we interpret the wins and losses we have in our day.

Positive mindset

The language we use to interpret the world has a huge impact on our behaviour.

Change your story

There are four levels of interpretation that our behaviour is based upon (we would like to acknowledge Martin Seligman's work in *Learned Optimism* as the original inspiration for this section):

- *regularity* — how often does that behaviour happen?
- *impact* — what is the impact of that behaviour on my life?
- *ownership* — who is responsible for that behaviour?
- *control* — what level of control do I have over that behaviour?

We have found that people trying to lose body fat fall down in these four levels of interpretation. They interpret their challenges and setbacks in an inaccurate, unrealistic and pessimistic way. In contrast, the people who are successful in losing body weight interpret their behaviours in an accurate, sensible and hopeful way.

Regularity — how often does that behaviour happen?

On the regularity spectrum we can have a behaviour that *always* happens at one end and a behaviour that *never* happens at the other, as shown in figure 14.1. This level looks at how we assign frequency to our behaviours.

Figure 14.1: the regularity spectrum

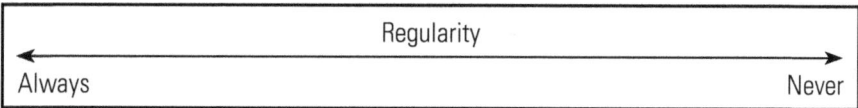

For example, some people make comments throughout their day such as, 'I am *always* late' or 'I *never* get through my work, there are *never* enough hours in a day!' Our behaviour tends to mimic our language, so declarative statements such as these can be quite dangerous and detrimental to our behaviour. We often hear people say, 'I never have any willpower', 'I always give up after three weeks into a health plan' and 'I'm hopeless, I can't say no to temptation'.

These sorts of statements can become self-fulfilling prophecies. To lose body fat we want to encourage a sense of regularity that is accurate, sensible and hopeful.

- *'I never have any willpower.'* A better statement is, 'In the past I have struggled to say no to temptation; however, I find it much easier when I have a clear goal and I know exactly what I am trying to achieve, like I do now'.

- *'I always give up after three weeks into a health plan.'* A better statement is, 'Previously I have tried different health fads and found them hard to stick to. The reason is that they were far too extreme and the change was too much to handle. However, my new plan is realistic and when I have a clear plan to follow I always stick to it'.

- *'I'm hopeless, I cannot say no to temptation.'* A better statement is, 'When I am around food that is not part of my eating plan I find it hard not to eat it. However, I know that saying no to it will help me achieve my goal and I will feel better about myself than if I cave in and eat that food'.

Be careful when making very broad statements about how regularly a behaviour occurs. Our internal dialogue greatly affects our behaviour. Therefore, if we continually tell ourselves something, negative or positive, our behaviour will begin to reflect it.

Impact — what is the impact of that behaviour on my life?

On the impact spectrum we can simply have a behaviour that has a *big* impact at one end and a behaviour that has a *little* impact at the other, as shown in figure 14.2. This level looks at how significant an impact we rate things to have.

Figure 14.2: the impact spectrum

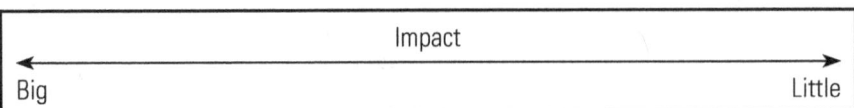

Throughout our day we can be dramatic and tend to exaggerate the impact of certain events. We miss the bus and we say to ourselves, 'It's just going to be one of those days'. Or we have a piece of cake at work and think, 'I have just ruined my diet'. When it comes to weight loss out of the four levels of interpretation we often see people interpret *impact* in the worst way. They go out on Friday night and overeat. They interpret this by saying, 'Well, that's ruined the weekend. There I go again, stuffing it up. I might as well forget about my weight loss plan. I guess I'll have to start again on Monday'.

A more accurate, sensible and hopeful way of interpreting this is 'Okay, I slipped up there, but it's only one meal out of 21 in the week. Sure it was fun to have a blow out but upon reflection it wasn't worth it. I need to remember that for next time. I'll just get back on the program and I'll walk for an extra hour to make up for it tomorrow morning. Everyone has a slip up from time to time. Don't focus on it — just get back on track'.

On the flip side, sometimes underestimating the impact of our behaviour can be the reason we never achieve any results. If we underestimate the impact of continually breaking our eating plan and skipping our exercise, we are never going to get the results we want. Statements like 'It's okay, I only ate half the block of chocolate' or 'I'm too tired to exercise today, I think I'll skip it' are not okay.

When trying to implement any weight loss program we must interpret the impact of our behaviour in an accurate, sensible and hopeful way.

Ownership — who is responsible for that behaviour?

On the ownership spectrum we simply have a behaviour that is due to *me* at one end and a behaviour that is due to *others* at the other, as shown in figure 14.3. This level looks at who influenced the final behaviour the most.

Figure 14.3: the ownership spectrum

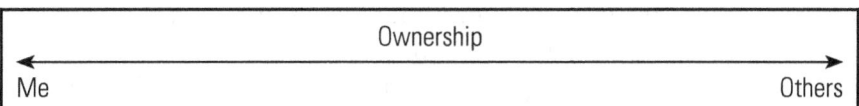

Often we outsource blame for certain behaviours rather than taking ownership of them. 'I had to have some birthday cake because they would be offended if I didn't.' 'Everyone around me was drinking wine, so I had to as well. I didn't want to stand out.' 'I ate the chocolate because I was tired and hungry. I have to have chocolate in the house for the kids. They get upset if we don't have it.'

A common thing we see is that people don't take responsibility for their actions. They try to outsource it to other people or situations. The higher people rate towards the 'me' end of the ownership spectrum, the more successful they will be with their weight loss.

Control — what level of control do I have over that behaviour?

On the control spectrum we can perceive that we have a *high* amount of control at one end and a *low* amount of control at the other, as shown in figure 14.4. This level looks at how much perceived control we have over our behaviour.

Figure 14.4: the control spectrum

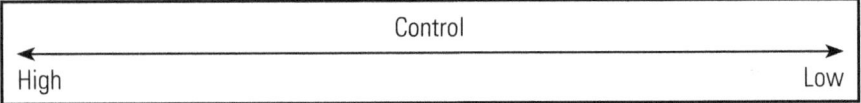

We have found that the higher people rate themselves on the level of control the more successful they are. Why? Because their interpretation of their behaviour is one area where they can control the outcome of their behaviour.

Often we hear people say 'I didn't do well this week because I was busy at work' or 'I had to travel this week'. People who rely on these statements are outsourcing blame for their behaviour to others. We found that the people who were really successful at losing body fat would come into our sessions and make statements like 'I went to a dinner that was mostly deep-fried finger food. I told the kitchen that I had some food allergies and asked if I could get a serve of vegetables. I could tell they weren't too happy but they did it anyway'.

While situations like these are not ideal, these people take control of their circumstances and get a better result. The more we believe that we are in control of our behaviour, the more likely we are to stick to any weight loss plan. When life gets in the way, the key is to focus on what we can control rather than not control and choose the appropriate behaviour.

* * *

How do we use all of this in the Good Enough Diet? When you are pursuing your new weight loss objective be very observant of how you interpret events, challenges and victories. In particular, keep in mind the four levels of interpretation. Aim at always ensuring that your interpretations are accurate, sensible and hopeful.

Takeaway tips

- Emotion is the most powerful controller of our behaviour. We are driven by emotions.
- The emotion we attach to something will determine how motivated we are to do something about it.
- Use the strategies outlined in this chapter to alter your exercise experience so you attach positive emotions to it.
- Realise that when we start exercising we can go through an initial period of discomfort before we begin to enjoy it.

Chapter 15

IT'S OKAY TO BE FAT

You have probably read the title of this chapter and thought how irresponsible we are as health professionals to think that it's okay to be fat. Do we believe it? Yes. But we're not suggesting a fat pride movement and sticking our heads in the sand about the health risks of obesity. Being overweight causes health risks — period. You would have to have been hiding under a rock if you were unaware of this. What we are arguing about is that discrimination against overweight people or fatism is not making the problem any better. It is making it worse. This not only goes for the discrimination against overweight people by other people, but the discrimination and self-loathing that overweight people dish out on themselves. It's amazing how many people talk to themselves in a way they wouldn't ever dare to talk to another person — regardless of whether it were their worst enemy.

Times are a-changin'

Fifty years ago, it was not okay to be a woman. Forty years ago, it was not okay to be black. Twenty years ago, it was not okay to be gay. To say that it was okay to be a woman/black/gay at the height of discrimination against these groups would have caused as much controversy as saying *'It's okay to be fat'* in today's society. In the Western world today, discriminating against fat people is the only socially acceptable form of discrimination in our society. Sure, discrimination still exists in other areas; however, it's not tolerated like fatism is.

Society judges people who are overweight as if they are in control of their weight. Truth be known, we are in control of many things, but we are not in control of the physiology that determines our body shape, size and storage. Although we are theoretically in control of what we eat, and how much we exercise, we cannot control physiological aspects of our metabolism, hormones or genes. With training, we can change our responses to taste or hunger that were developed from childhood, but we have to work at these like any skill or type of personal development.

Being obese, with a body mass index (BMI) of between 30 and 35, has been shown to reduce a person's longevity by about three years. Interestingly enough, being underweight has been shown to reduce longevity by even more years. Compare this with happiness. It has been shown that being unhappy can reduce your longevity by over nine years. We contribute to the unhappiness of people (and ourselves) who are overweight by unfairly judging their character according to their weight. The truth is that we all have issues. Some of us wear our issues on the inside and some of us wear our issues on the outside. If you wear them on the outside, you need to know that this doesn't reflect your character. You do have the willpower, you do have the strength and you do have all the resources available inside you to make a change. The more you beat up on yourself, the more you will self-sabotage your efforts.

A shift in perspective

When we discussed the concept that it's okay to be fat with others, the initial reaction was always 'But, it's not okay to be fat', followed by 'People need to be aware that they have a problem, so they can fix it'. Now this is just ridiculous. After treating over 10 000 people in clinics, working with thousands more in seminars, listening to other health professionals and just general chit chat between our friends and colleagues, we know one thing. Most, if not all, women who are overweight are fully aware of the fact. They may not tell you this every time they see you, but they know that they are fat. In fact, many people who are nowhere near overweight also think that they are fat. How many women do you know who are still dieting at 60 years of age and will tell you how gorgeous they were at 30 (with hindsight), but when they were 30, thought they were fat? Interestingly, while women overestimate their size, men have been shown to do the opposite and underestimate their weight.

Yes, it's true that if people decide to lose weight, they need to be aware of their situation and the issues. However, we would argue that people who are overweight have moved past the awareness, information and desire stages of message buy-in and need assistance with the 'how' of weight loss, not the 'why' of weight loss. There is much evidence to show that people think they are more overweight than they actually are, and being unaware of their situation is extremely rare.

Just like telling kids they are dumb won't make them smarter, telling someone they are fat won't make them thinner. In fact, research in intelligence shows us that the more we tell a child they are dumb, or that they are from a disadvantaged group, the lower their IQ scores or examination results will be. Telling someone (particularly children) they are fat actually increases their likelihood of binge eating and emotional eating rather than motivating them to do something about their weight. This applies equally to you when you are considering telling yourself how fat you are, too. It is so hard to see someone you love or see yourself put on an unhealthy amount of weight. If you have told someone more than once — they know. Instead, focus on what you can control, such as removing temptations, creating exercise opportunities and eating healthily as we've described within this book, rather than nagging your loved ones about their weight and the consequences of obesity.

There is a big difference in knowing that you're okay and believing you're okay. Knowing you deserve better and believing you deserve better. Knowing you can do it and believing you can do it. Many self-help books will tell you that you need to change your beliefs. However, this is unlikely to happen in the time you have to lose weight. If your self-perception is that you are fat, even when you are thin, you will believe you are fat. What if believing that you are fat is okay, that fat was just a descriptive word like 'blonde' or 'brunette' without the good or bad attached to it? Accepting this belief as a neutral belief will allow you to live life to the fullest.

Diane's story

In our clinics, many people want to lose a certain amount of weight. The consultation for many is different but the pain is the same. Diane was one of Tara's favourite clients. She had just turned 40 when we first met and owned a successful marketing and PR consultancy. She arrived at the Health Management office as bright as can be, a smile from ear to ear. Even though she was not obese, at 86 kilograms, she was a little overweight. This was causing her pain. As much as she tried to hide the pain with her outgoing personality, infectious enthusiasm and wide smile, Tara could feel it.

When she came into Tara's office, after the introductions were complete, she told her why she was there.

'I want to be 65 kilograms!' she declared, like she had been thinking about it for months.

'Have you ever been 65 kilograms before?' Tara asked.

'Yes, this was the weight I was when I was 26, the year I was married', she beamed proudly.

'Great, so do you think you'll be happy at 65 kilograms? Do you think this is a good weight?' Tara asked.

'Yes, definitely. If I am 65 kilograms, I will be healthy, I will be happy, gosh I was attractive at that weight—oh, let me show you', Diane exclaimed as she quickly whipped out her iPhone and proceeded to show Tara photos she had scanned into Facebook when she was her 'perfect' weight.

Diane did look gorgeous, for her height, 65 kilograms was quite lean, and she looked very athletic. Tara wanted to know a little more about this weight and how Diane felt about it. So she asked her, 'Okay Diane, tell me, how did you feel at this weight? How did you feel before your wedding, on your honeymoon and on the special day?' At this point, the everpresent big smile faded from Diane's face, the creases near

> her temples flattened and her eyes started to well with tears. She was completely quiet. She looked at Tara, and it was like half of her wished she'd never made the appointment and the other half wished she would just disappear. 'Ummm', she stammered, 'I thought I was fat then too ... I was gorgeous and I thought I was fat'.

So now we have to ask ourselves is a person better off being thin and thinking they are fat, or being fat and thinking they are okay? And does the mere issue of thinking you are fat when you are thin make you fat?

Acceptance of self, regardless of weight, is one of the necessary stages of weight loss and maintenance. Without this, people will self-sabotage and punish themselves through weight gain.

Self-talk and support

Diane's story is not a one-off. If you have a specific weight in mind that you would like to be, think about what you thought of yourself when you were that weight. If you have always thought that you were fat, it's not just your weight we need to change, but your thoughts about yourself, so that when you are at a healthy weight, you stop beating up on yourself. This is one of the major keys in ensuring your weight loss is sustainable.

As we have said before, knowing that you are okay with your weight is different from believing that you really are okay. Although you may never believe you are okay, accepting this thought as okay is the key to happiness with self and ultimately a much needed strategy in good enough weight loss and maintenance.

Your self-talk becomes your reality, so it is important to practise talking to yourself positively. It is best to talk to yourself out loud or write down what you want to believe. At the start, you may feel silly saying this to yourself — you may even feel like you are lying. However, over time you will believe what you are saying and this will put you in a more positive space to accept compliments. When we have developed low self-esteem, we find it difficult to receive compliments. It is like we put a mirror up when someone compliments us and the compliments bounce off us like they never happened. When we are told something negative, we turn the mirror around towards us and it amplifies these negative feelings.

If you find that you do this, practise mirror affirmations before you go to bed. The process is simple, but it may feel awkward at first. Look in the mirror each night before bed and say three positive affirmations. Positive affirmations can be things that you are grateful for about yourself; things that you liked about yourself on that day; things that are your strengths; or things you plan to do. If you can't think of anything, that's easy, remember a compliment that someone paid you recently and use that to begin with. Even if you start off not believing what you say about yourself, you will still enjoy the benefits. Over time, you will believe what you are saying — and in many cases the positive affirmations are truth. Over time, your self-esteem will improve. We know that those with better self-esteem and value are less likely to self-sabotage, fall off their dieting or exercise routine, or regain lost weight.

Finding a team that is supportive, yet nag free, is helpful in keeping your accountability and staying on track when you feel like giving up. This may or may not be your partner and/or health professionals. Choose those you want in your team, rather than feeling like everyone has to be supportive. Some people just nag and don't understand. Find a group of people — those who are in your area or that you can chat with over the phone, or even via the internet — and enlist them to help you achieve your goals.

Always remember that we are all different. What works for others may not work for you and vice versa. This doesn't mean that you ignore all advice from others, just make sure that you critically evaluate it.

Takeaway tips

- Change your attitude towards your weight.
- Remember, your weight status doesn't say anything about your personal attributes.
- Say three positive things to yourself in the mirror nightly before bed.
- Enlist a great team who will support you through the tough times and the good times.
- Keep to your guns when you know something is right for you and it makes sense.
- Remember that self-sabotaging doesn't hurt anyone but you.
- Know and believe that it's okay to be fat.

Chapter 16

EXERCISE AND THE THIRD SPACE

Work–life balance research shows us that the more we can go home, turn off from work and not think about it, the less stressed and the better our relationships will be. We will also be more refreshed and creative the next day when we return to work. However, turning off from work is difficult. One of the reasons why this is challenging is that during the day we build up stress hormones in our brains, things like adrenaline and cortisol. When we have these coursing through our brain we tend to be more aggressive, impulsive, emotionally volatile and blow things out of proportion. The beautiful thing about exercise is that it uses up these hormones, leaving us feeling refreshed, calm and with clarity of thought. Therefore, we can use exercise to improve our work–life balance.

A concept that Adam developed is called the 'third space'. He first discovered this concept when he was managing the health of a high-profile Australian businessman who clearly had a lot going on in his life and had a high degree of stress.

The third space

Adam arrived at the businessman's home for their first meeting at 7.30 pm. What Adam immediately noticed about him was that he was incredibly relaxed, calm, engaged, fun and energetic. Adam thought, 'Oh, that's how I want to be when I get home'.

Once they had finished the session, Adam said, 'I hope this isn't out of line but how do you go from psycho businessman to super dad?' The businessman replied, 'Well, I used to get it very wrong. Previously I would walk in the door, I would finish my wife's sentences because she didn't talk fast enough, I would yell at my kids because they weren't efficient with the time they had available. It got to the point where I came home one day and as I opened the door the kids scattered. It broke my heart. I thought what sort of a jerk am I? My kids don't even want to see me at the end of the day. When I sat down to think about it I realised that I was this hurricane that tore through the house and left a trail of destruction behind me. I thought desperate times call for desperate measures. So I built a new entrance into the house [hmmm, we realise not all of us have the cashflow to do this, but read on] with a doorway that goes from the garage to my bedroom. I get home, go through this doorway and straight into my room without talking to anyone in the family. The first thing I do is have a shower, then I come out and get dressed in casual clothes, and then I do a visualisation/relaxation exercise that lasts for about four minutes. Then I go out to greet the family. I lose 15 to 20 minutes, but the mindset I am in is worth every minute lost. In that time I think about how I want to be when I go out to greet the family, how I want to act, how I want to feel and how I want to make them feel'.

Adam was impressed with the technique that the businessman used to 'decompress' after work and decided to call this ritual the 'third space'.

Adam has used this 'third space' technique with great success over the years with many people to improve their transition between work and home. However, what he has found is that when this third space includes exercise, it greatly improves how people behave when they return home and walk through the door, for the simple reason that exercise reduces stress, anxiety and anger, leaving you in a much better space to interact with your family.

A great example of this is when Adam was completing a consulting job with Shane, a manager of a call centre in Tasmania. Shane had a mild heart attack while Adam was consulting there. When Shane was well enough to return to work Adam told him about the third space concept. He suggested that Shane use exercise as his third space to improve his heart function but also to help him wind down after work. Adam met up with Shane eight and a half months later and asked him how his third space was going. Shane replied, 'I haven't missed a day since you told me about it'. Adam was stunned! 'That is amazing! Your motivation must be incredible', he said. 'Oh no, motivation has nothing to do with it, as soon as I get in the door my wife grabs my bag, hands me my raincoat and says, "On your way". I am in such a good mood after my walk that she won't let me miss it. Actually, it has really improved the relationship I have with my family. The only problem is that July in Tassie is absolutely freezing, horizontal rain hits me in the face as I open the door, and my wife is pushing me in the back saying, "You'll be okay, off you go".'

Ask the average person what they would like more of and work–life balance is always high on their list. When you ask them what balance would look like, they often say, 'Well, I would have more time with my friends and family'. However, time is not the right measure of work–life balance. There are many people who are at home with their family but the only time they interact with them is grunting if someone gets in the way of the TV. Balance is about the quality of the interaction you have with the people in your life. What underpins the quality of the interaction you have with the people you live with is how you show up when you walk through the door. If you come in angry, frustrated or disinterested, you have set yourself up for a disastrous interaction, no matter how nice you are after this first impression. If you are optimistic, invigorated and enthusiastic when you walk through the door, you are setting yourself up for the best possible interaction.

In the rest of this chapter we discuss tips on making exercise and the third space part of your life.

Exercise on your way home

Research has shown that many gym members don't actually live anywhere near their gym. The gym just happens to be on their way home. This is a good strategy for two reasons.

1. If you go home first and then try to go out and exercise, the chance of your leaving the house is very, very small, particularly if you have a family, as they will want your time and they will want to interact with you. Also, there are always things to do when you get home, such as preparing dinner and cleaning up. Finally, there is the fact that after a long day at work as soon as your butt hits the lounge, it's very unlikely that you'll want to get up for the rest of the evening.
2. It leverages the concept of the third space and helps you improve your mood and reduce your physical tension, before you greet your family.

Give the pets some love

Since the reduction of free time, a concerning new trend is the rise of obesity and diabetes in dogs. This is happening because their owners are too busy to walk them. A great strategy for losing weight yourself is to grab the dog and take it for a quick walk straight after you get in the door. The combination of exercise and the unconditional love from your dog can't be beaten when it comes to lifting your mood after a long day at work.

Team sport

When we think about the impact of working too much on relationships, we invariably think of romantic relationships. However, studies are indicating that our interpersonal relationships (friendships) are suffering due to our fast-paced world. A great way of seeing friends and dropping a couple of extra kilos is by organising an after-work team sport. Whether it is netball, basketball, touch football or even a dance class, the combination of seeing your friends, having some fun and incorporating high-intensity exercise will have you on cloud nine when you return home and walk through the door.

Make it part of the commute

Road rage is on the rise due to traffic congestion. Public transport can be a challenge, with late services and being squashed into a small space with smelly, sweaty people. All of these factors can leave you feeling downright annoyed when you get home. Attempt to slot physical activity into your commute. If you live close to your workplace, obviously you could ride or walk to work. If public transport is part of your commute, time permitting aim to walk home from the bus stop or train station.

Segment your life

Even if you don't have family, creating a third space allows you to shut off the emotional energy from work, and will leave you feeling more energised at home and better equipped to deal with the following day.

Takeaway tips

- People often take the baggage of a tough day at work home with them, which affects their interactions with their family.
- The third space is the transitional gap between work and home.
- Create your own third space to help you with the transition from work to home.
- Use exercise as your third space, a time to debrief with yourself, create closure and open up space for your next interaction. Exercise improves your brain chemistry and elevates your mood.
- Stop at the gym or pool on your way home from a tough day or meeting.
- Go for a walk as soon as you get home after work.
- Work–life balance is about how you 'show up' and the quality of the interactions you have with the people in your life, not how much time you have with them.
- Use this gap to think about how you will 'show up', what sort of mood you will you be in when you walk through the door and if you want to share that with them.
- Remember, it is not when you show up, but how you show up.

Chapter 17

It's okay to be hungry

If you are walking around the supermarket, playground, theme park or, in fact, anywhere that is densely populated with parents and children, what is the most common phrase you hear? That's right — it's unmistakable. 'Muuuum — I'm hungry.' To this, more often than not mums in unison around the world will pull out their carefully packed, brightly coloured Tupperware containers with their child's name taped across the translucent plastic.

This often happens in our clinics. We are not suggesting you starve your children, but surely a 30-minute dietitian or exercise physiology appointment doesn't warrant a packed lunch.

As babies we cry when we are hungry, we cry because we cannot speak and we only eat when we are hungry. As children get older, parents continue to see being hungry as a negative feeling — emotion even — and want to fix this straight away. Our parents subconsciously remember the helplessness they felt when you cried as a baby, and try the first thing that they know might take away your pain. The problem is that by the time we are toddlers or small children, we realise that food not only fixes hunger, it also fixes boredom. Because we can't get our own food, it means that mum or dad will have to stop what they are doing and give us some more attention. Last but not least — some food tastes so yummy. As you can see, as a child there is a lot of pay-off by saying that we're hungry.

As we get older, hunger continues to be one of those things that we try to ward off. Diet plan after diet plan promises a hunger-free solution, and this reassures us. Now, there is one thing that you need to know — feeling hungry is not necessarily a bad thing. It's okay to be hungry.

Naturally thin people can go out and feel hungry, but they can wait till the next meal or until they get home before they eat. People who are at the more overweight end of the scale can't wait. When they get hungry, they need to eat something to tide them over to the next meal. Often, the problem is that the snacks chosen usually add up to more daily kilojoules than the meals you eat, so you effectively double up.

Don't fill the space

Some people will tell you to eat something like vegetable sticks or low kilojoule snack bars to prevent you from overeating. Truth is, you will probably still overeat, and will always need something immediately when you feel a slight hunger pang. Eating low kilojoule snacks is a bandaid situation, and although eating more veggies is not a bad thing for your weight, we want to get to the cause of the problem.

What we want you to do is to start getting comfortable with feeling hungry. This isn't something that will happen immediately after you put down this book. Like all habits, it is something that takes time to develop.

It is interesting when you watch children at school. They (usually) don't get hungry until the lunch bell reminds them that it's food time and when the final bell of the day signals home time. However, on weekends they become eating machines. It seems like they are hungry every five minutes.

Conditioned to eat

If we had a cutest client competition in our clinic, Madeline Jones would take the prize hands down. Her smile used to light up the office and her positive, inquisitive and friendly attitude would turn the worst day around—for us, for our staff and for our clients waiting with her. She was classified as morbidly obese for her height and age, but that didn't stop her from participating in school sports, dancing and playing with her friends.

Maddy liked to be the centre of attention and had more friends than fingers and toes. On weekends, she would go and play at her grandparents' house and she was the apple of their eyes. When we chatted to George, her grandpa, he admitted that he just couldn't say no when she said she was hungry—and she said she was hungry a lot. George used to keep special fun food for Maddy, because he knew she liked it. At home after school, the same thing happened and she would eat all afternoon until dinner time and still polish off her plate.

Maddy had lost what it felt like to be hungry. When we asked her what hungry felt like, the feelings she described had nothing to do with her tummy—the feelings she described were of boredom or feeling neglected (although the reality of her situation was far from this, as Maddy liked to be the centre of attention all the time). To help Maddy we set up a system of conditioning her hunger so it was more appropriate.

Maddy's lunchbox was split into three sections—little lunch bell, big lunch bell and after school bell. She would eat her afternoon snack while waiting for her mum, Teagan, to pick her up from school. The dinner bell made a return appearance in the Jones household, and this would ring at dinner time and when it was time for a healthy dessert. Teagan found this the hardest and would call us for support. She felt like a bad mother, like she was starving Maddy. We would reassure her that eating six times a day was enough for a six year old and that she was building the healthy foundations for Maddy's future.

> ### Conditioned to eat (cont'd)
>
> For the first couple of weeks Maddy would kick, scream and cry about being hungry, which, in a society where food is love, would break Teagan's heart. We encouraged Teagan to replace food with real displays of love — hugs, kisses, reassurance and playing with Maddy. The same tactic was used at Maddy's grandparents' on the weekends, with similar initial results. The bell was rung at the same times that the school bells rang. We used techniques such as serving the recommended amount of food on a plate, practising slow eating and chewing, and sitting at the table, which all helped Maddy to cope with her lowered food intake. Because she was a child, we didn't want Maddy to lose too much weight; we wanted it to go down very slowly while her height caught up with her weight.
>
> Two years later, Maddy was the same happy girl, still on the higher end of the growth charts, but within them nonetheless. She didn't need the bells anymore to remind her when it was the appropriate time to eat, but also didn't feel restricted. Teagan still speaks of how bad she felt when restricting food from Maddy, but is now so glad that she did.

Now, you may not have children, but you may have an inner child just like Maddy. We found that many of our clients had the same issue. They didn't know what true hunger was and were guided by external hunger rather than internal hunger — hunger that comes from the head, taste buds or heart rather than hunger that comes from the belly. With Maddy, although it was hard, change was helped by her supportive mother and grandparents. When you are trying to get yourself to recognise appropriate hunger cues, you need to be disciplined by sticking to the rules, and limit the internal negotiation.

There are a couple of ways to do this. Some of our clients found it helpful to think of their inner child and be the carer for the innocent child inside them that they are trying to re-establish appropriate food behaviour with. This works especially well for parents. Set up the rules of behaviour. The times you are able to eat will be based on whether you are a hungry eater (maximum of four times a day) or whether you are fine with your portion sizes (maximum of six times per day). Remember that liquid kilojoules also count as food.

Embracing hunger

After you have set out your meal times, embracing hunger is the next step. The more you focus on it, the hungrier you will feel. You need to acknowledge your hunger, determine whether it is head, heart, taste bud or belly hunger, and then acknowledge that it's okay to feel hungry. If you are at home or in a private place, a helpful tip is to acknowledge this out loud, 'I feel hungry, my hunger is coming from my belly, and it's okay to feel like this'. The first couple of times you do this, you will give in and head to the fridge or closest store and buy something. Again, this is something you need to stick to for it to become long lasting. Try again the next time you feel hungry and over time you will become comfortable with this sensation, and the negative feelings associated with feeling hungry will diminish. You will also find that head, heart and taste bud hunger will not haunt you anymore.

Once you have developed an eating schedule and you're acknowledging that it's okay to be hungry, it's time to practise behaviours that will normalise your hunger response.

You should wake up hungry. Not starving, but hungry. Going eight hours without food should allow you to wake up feeling like you can eat something. This is a major reason why people tell us that they don't eat breakfast. Now for the hard truth. If you are not hungry when you wake up, you are either eating too much the previous day, and especially the previous night, or you are eating too late in the day.

Not eating within two hours of going to bed is the first step to resolve this, and the second step is eating small portions at your evening meals. As we have said numerous times throughout this book, half of your plate should contain non-starchy vegetables, a small (about a cup, or fist size) serve of carbohydrates and a palm-hand-size serving of lean meat, chicken or fish. Unless you're an athlete or working physically all day, this is enough food for your evening meal. As we discussed in chapter 3, serving your meal on a plate makes you eat considerably less than if the food is served from bowls in the centre of the table. For very small children who are pretty good at regulating their food, this may have the opposite effect, so let them pick and choose how much they eat.

As well as serving food on a plate, research from the Cornell University Food and Brand Lab, headed by Professor Brian Wansink, author of *Mindless Eating: Why We Eat More Than We Think*, has shown that eating from a smaller plate than the platters that seem to have replaced dinner plates of late will reduce intake without making you feel deprived. Professor Wansink ran a series of experiments where the usual 27.5 centimetre (11 inch) diameter plate was replaced with a 22.5 centimetre (9 inch) diameter plate. At this size people ate less without realising it. When the plate was reduced to a diameter of 17.5 centimetres (7 inches), those who ate from these plates realised they were eating much less and felt hungry. These days it is quite difficult to find smaller plates; however, visits to op shops, secondhand shops or your grandma's cupboard will result in some great finds. If this isn't an option, you can order plates online from <www.mindlesseating.org>, which offers a range of plates, including our personal favourite — the compartment plate. It's not only the smaller size, but it has grooves to allow you to fill up half of the plate with non-starchy vegetables. An Australian version is available from <www.greatideas.net.au>.

Rebuilding your food foundations will also occur from eating more slowly. We are sure you have heard the statement that it takes 20 minutes for your stomach to tell your head that you're full. The whole process of eating should result in your feeling more full, so it's important to eat slowly and chew your food very well.

There are a couple of tricks you can do. You can chew your food and just when you would usually swallow, chew your food again. Don't watch television and don't use the internet or speak on the phone while you are eating. When you do these things you eat more quickly and don't chew your food as well. If you have ever eaten in an atmospheric Greek restaurant, you will also realise how fast music affects your eating speed, so if you have music on, keep it slow.

There are technology tools to retrain your eating, like the Nutrition Guru's Eating Trainer iPhone application. It has a 31-day program to help you retrain your eating and become more mindful, as well as a simple tool that signals when you should eat, and when you should put your knife and fork down. We recommend to our clients that they should put their knife and fork down (or food, if eating something like a wrap) between mouthfuls, cross their hands and chew their food well. They should pick up their knife and fork only after swallowing. By eating more slowly, the changes felt between being hungry and being full will be more obvious. You don't need to eat until you feel full, but until you feel satisfied. Many of our clients were amazed that this simple trick resulted in food being left on their plates for the first time in ages. The food left on your plate means kilojoules remain on the plate rather than on your body, and that is great news for weight loss.

The last tip that can be helpful in retraining your hunger and eating behaviour is to keep a food diary. Even if you are not showing this to anyone, we found that our clients who recorded what they were eating became more aware of what they put in their mouths. As health professionals, we know that when we ask someone what they eat, it comes out a little skewed. This is not because people lie, they just forget what they have eaten. Writing down what you've eaten immediately afterwards is helpful. You can do this on a sheet of paper, in a diary, or by using your phone. There are iPhone applications for recording your food, as well as a photo food diary, where you simply take a photo of your meals and at the end of the day you can email them to yourself and print them out, or you can email them directly to your dietitian/exercise physiologist/doctor — whoever is looking after your diet.

As you can see, getting back to eating well is not just about the food you eat or the exercise you do. It is important to acknowledge the things that hold us back, including hunger — whether it be true belly hunger or head, heart or taste bud hunger. Acknowledging that hunger is okay, and then setting up some steps so it is not in control of your eating, will make you the one that's in control, not your hunger.

Takeaway tips

- Acknowledge where your hunger is coming from — head, heart, taste bud or belly.
- Acknowledge that being hungry is okay.
- Remember food is not love. There are other ways to show yourself or others that you love them.
- Set specific times where you are 'allowed' to eat.
- Use smaller dinner plates — 22.5 centimetres (9 inches) in diameter.
- Serve meals on plates, rather than banquet style.

- Turn off technology at meal times.
- Play slow music during meals.
- Chew your food well.
- Eat slowly, and use strategies to help you do this.
- Record what you eat — written, typed or photographed.

Part IV GOOD ENOUGH MYTH-BUSTING

Chapter 18

DEMYSTIFYING MYTHS

When it comes to health information, for some reason we Australians like to believe that it simply can't be that easy. We like to take the hard road, and health professionals support us in doing so. The problem is that this sets us up for failure and then we give up and return to our old habits.

It seems the more difficult and lifestyle incompatible the proposed solution, the more we believe and follow the advice — for a short period anyway. When this is combined with the ease of accessible information from online sources, life can become overwhelming for those trying to lose weight.

The most important thing for you to know is that when you get to the stage where your weight and your life are on track, you will want to help others follow your path. This is what many authors, life coaches or 'experts' do. They profess to know the solutions to the world because *something* worked for them. On the television program *The Biggest Loser*, how many of the biggest losers have returned for the season's finale as a personal trainer? Yes, I, too, have lost count. Now, it's always good to hear from people who have been in your shoes, and come out of it in joggers; however, there is also danger in this approach. Just because something worked for someone, it doesn't mean it will work for you. And even if whatever they recommend does help you lose weight, it doesn't mean you will be healthier if you follow their advice. This is why throughout this book our advice is backed up by large research experiments that included tens of thousands of people. On top of this, we try the research out on our clients to make sure the conclusions are transferable to the real world.

We see the same mistakes made over and over, but we also understand that when you want to lose weight, it is only human nature that at first you will get excited and desperate for change to happen immediately.

Use your head

Ron and Nola had just retired and moved to the Sunshine Coast from Sydney for a seachange, a slower pace and a healthier lifestyle. Ron had kidney problems that were exacerbated by his weight and his doctor suggested that he see us to lose his excess kilos, especially from around his middle.

Ron and Nola's grandson, Jeff, had just taught Nola how to use the internet. Now this was the start of all the world of problems for us, as we were trying to get Ron to lose weight sensibly and carefully without negatively affecting his kidneys or creating other health issues.

Ron loved to play golf and his mates at the golf club were like a group of 15-year-old school girls sharing stories of how to lose weight as quickly as possible, while Nola was finding all sorts of weird and wonderful weight loss information on the internet to give to Ron. The issue was that Ron and Nola didn't have the understanding about how to seek information on the internet discerningly and didn't know what to look out for to avoid getting misleading advice when it came to dieting.

Each week our sessions would deviate from making real change to clarifying misconceptions and dispelling myths. In the end we taught Ron and Nola how to properly assess information, which gave them some power to make their own choices and at the same time reassured us that they were making informed choices.

Mistakes we make

The mistakes we see vary, but a few pop up more than others. One mistake we see people making over and over again is getting advice that is essentially ideal, but that either isn't practical for their lifestyle or doesn't align with their values. We have had vegetarians trying to follow high protein, low carbohydrate diets, which just isn't very nutritious.

Another common mistake is to rely on the advice of a neighbour or another poorly qualified person on what worked for them/their friend/their mother. It's rather alarming but we have found that even some doctors do this. For example, for some patients with particular bowel conditions, pregnancy multivitamins are the best type of vitamins to take because they are higher in zinc, iron, calcium and omega-3 fats. However, this is true for a specific patient with specific bowel conditions. One day, Tara advised a GP who had a bowel condition to take these multivitamins. With the best intentions, this GP started telling all of his patients, with or without bowel conditions, to start taking pregnancy multivitamins. Not a huge issue, but an example where even smart, well-educated people who understand the body give advice to others that may not be right for them.

Media outlets such as television, the radio, magazines and newspapers round off the list for sources of easy, yet possibly not always the most accurate, weight loss information. However, without a doubt, the most problematic source of weight loss information these days is the internet. A quick look at the Google keyword tool shows us that each month there are 7.5 million searches for weight loss, which means 90 million per year! It's true that there is a lot of excellent information on the internet, but there is just as much unreliable information. Some of the worst websites are created by people with good intentions, who are misinformed themselves. Other websites are set up by people wanting to make a quick buck by selling bogus programs or products with no concern for the problems they could be causing people who take their shonky advice.

Be discerning

If you are seeking reliable and accurate information, it is crucial that you are discerning about the promises given on programs or websites. Just today we received an e-newsletter promoting a new 'scientifically proven' weight loss program. After scanning the attached website, which also offered the same claims, we decided to call the company to see what research had been done to prove these claims. The young woman who answered the phone couldn't verify any research, but said that we could be assured that the program was scientifically proven if we wanted to lose weight. Obviously we asked to speak to someone else, who told us that 'the research was commercial intellectual property' — code for not scientific evidence. From the response we received, it was obvious that they had never been questioned about this statement in their advertising, which is surprising, as we expected at least a prepared statement from them.

Although there are set regulations for both food and weight loss companies about what they can advertise, the sheer number of companies, websites, products and services available makes these regulations difficult to police. On top of this, if these companies and websites are based overseas, they are governed by different laws from those in Australia.

When assessing information to see whether it is credible, check the following.

- Is the website run by a private company or a credible association, such as the Heart Foundation, Diabetes Australia or Dietitians Association of Australia?

- If the website is a company, what are the qualifications of the authors? Check for qualification clarification rather than simply a title such as 'nutritionist' or 'weight loss coach', as anyone can use any title they like.

- Determine what the information is trying to sell. If it is based around a product, it is probably skewed.

- If there is reference to research, is the research indicated on the website or another available source?

- Avoid being tempted by testimonials as these can be made up, or are not typical results.

- Does the advice align with your lifestyle and values?

- Is the advice for weight loss rather than health?

- Does the advice promise unbelievable results?

- Does the program include a number of pills and potions?

📌 Does the program, service or product claim to cure cancer or diabetes or something similar?

Once you have checked these things, you will be able to more accurately assess whether information is credible or not. In our work the most important question we ask ourselves when given new information is 'Does this make sense physiologically?', which means does it make sense with how we know the body to work and how the body absorbs nutrients?

Too good to be true

As well as the dodgy myths fuelled by commercial interests, there are also some myths that are created by scientific evidence — conclusions that are great in the lab but not always applicable to the real world, or misinterpreted by the media and/or health professionals.

A few years ago, a brilliant research paper was published claiming that chocolate milk was more beneficial as a rehydration beverage for cyclists than a sports drink. It claimed that because of the combination of protein, sugar and salt, a group of cyclists who drank chocolate milk instead of a specifically designed sports drink actually performed better than the group who consumed the sports drink. The media grabbed onto this with two hands and consequently the conclusions were blasted over radio waves and featured in newspapers around the country.

At the time, Tara was working as a sports dietitian and was helping a number of cyclists improve their sporting performance. Unfortunately, the media reports reached her cyclists before she could and, before she knew it, her team was taking chocolate milk along with them on their long rides. Yes, that's right, they took chocolate milk in a drinks bottle on their four-hour rides in the blazing hot sun — chocolate milk?! As you can imagine, this experiment didn't translate well in practice. Tara's cyclists did consume chocolate milk during their rides, but it was purchased about halfway along their ride, rather than taken with them.

Overall, if something sounds too good to be true — it probably is. There is a blank cheque awaiting the company that invents the magic weight loss pill or potion. And pharmaceutical companies are spending millions of dollars trying to develop such a drug — one that helps us lose weight, keep it off and be accompanied with minimal side effects, so you can understand that something that genuinely works to lose weight is not going to bought off the internet for $50 or even $500.

The Good Enough Diet is about doing what counts and forgetting the stuff that wastes physical and emotional time. Yes, we understand that there is a placebo effect when you take pills and potions; however, we want you to stop self-sabotaging yourself by wasting your time and emotional energy looking for and trying out fads. There is an opportunity cost to this. Remember your balance bar graph that we discussed in this book's introduction? You could be spending that wasted time on your physical health or other areas of your life that were revealed to be important by this graph.

Takeaway tips

- Don't believe everything you read or hear.
- Just because it is right for you, doesn't mean it is right for everyone.
- Question statements like 'scientifically proven' or 'clinical results' and look for back-up evidence.
- Be discerning when looking at weight loss options on the internet, or for that matter on television, radio or in print media.
- Be aware of the context of scientific research to ensure it applies to your life in the real world and if it will work for you.
- Don't waste emotional time on trying to find a quick fix, it is just one way to self-sabotage your success.

Chapter 19

FOOD COMBINING

One question we are commonly asked is whether or not it is unhealthy to combine different foods and eat them together in one meal. Some fad diets suggest you eat fruit on its own, while other weight loss programs suggest that you avoid eating protein foods such as meat, chicken or fish with carbohydrate foods such as pasta, bread, rice or potato.

In the Good Enough Diet what we want you to do is combine these foods for the exact same reason that the those weight loss programs suggest that you separate them. If you eat protein and carbohydrate foods together, the nutrients are absorbed more slowly than if you eat those foods separately. If eaten together, the nutrients, along with the energy, are digested more slowly, thus providing longer-lasting energy levels throughout the day.

The 3.30 pm energy slump

Jacqui Rickard has always found 3.30 pm hard. By this time she is tired, easily irritated and craving something sweet. This would be fine if Jacqui didn't have any responsibilities, but she does. She is the Human Resources manager at a major financial institution and therefore needs to be on the top of her game at all times. At 52 years of age, she is just starting to go through her change of life, and her only child, Sarah, is now a beautiful young married woman.

Jacqui has battled with her weight for as long as she can remember, but can always pinpoint midafternoon as her dieting downfall. Even when she used to pick Sarah up from school, Jacqui would find herself wolfing down similar snacks to her athletic daughter, even though she was sitting in front of a computer or in meetings for most of the day while Sarah's day consisted of nonstop energy burning. Besides her afternoon treat — if you can call it that — Jacqui's meals are what seem to be relatively healthy. She eats cereal, milk and fruit for breakfast, a low-fat cereal bar for morning tea, a salad sandwich for lunch, rice crackers or fruit for afternoon tea, meat with three vegetables for dinner, and/or dessert, in which fruit and yoghurt are on the menu. Jacqui always chooses low-fat foods when she can, and particularly ones with diet branding, because she assumes a dietitian or nutritionist has created them, so they will be good for her.

Jacqui's story is typical for men and women from the baby boomer and generation X eras, who grew up when there was a strong focus on low-fat foods, with myriad products arriving on the market sporting this claim. Since then more snack food has become available, and although it is low in fat, even if the carbohydrate content hasn't been increased, the kilojoule count could be much lower. These foods are also highly processed, so the nutrients and energy are absorbed more quickly, increasing insulin responses, and this combined with excess blood sugar equals increased storage of fat.

> Jacqui had been convinced that these foods were healthy for her to eat, and for some, this may be true. However, because she was still putting on weight, and particularly feeling tired and irritable in the afternoon, we needed to try a new strategy. After looking at her diet, we could see that it was slightly too high in kilojoules to lose weight, and even without the treats in the afternoon, her portions had to reduce. But eating small, regular portions of a high-carbohydrate, low-fat and low-protein food diet was making Jacqui get hungry quite quickly. This is not unusual, and because this type of diet is commonly seen as the healthy way to eat, Jacqui was only one of our many clients who experienced similar problems.

If you are also like Jacqui, you will find that you can't seem to feel full with a reasonable amount of food and end up eating a lot more than you need. You may feel tired or starving between 3.00 pm and 4.30 pm, even though you have had all of your meals for the day. You might find that you just don't have the energy levels that you used to have. Finally, you might find that despite your best efforts, your weight continues to sit where it is, even though you are eating low-fat and have started exercising.

If this is you, you need to pay closer attention to how you eat foods and ensure you combine your proteins with your carbohydrate foods.

Successful food combining

Foods contain a mixture of what we call macronutrients. These are the nutrients that give us energy, and you will know them as protein, carbohydrate and fat. Different food groups are usually more dominant in one type of macronutrient than another will be. For example, breads and cereals are high in carbohydrates, meats are high in protein and fruit is high in carbohydrate. Dairy and legumes contain moderate amounts of both protein and carbohydrate, except for cheese, which is protein dominant. Depending on the food and how it is served will determine the fat content.

When combining nutrients, we should take notice of the carbohydrate and protein content of foods and try to eat them together.

There is benefit to eating meals that contain moderate amounts of carbohydrate and protein and small amounts of fat. The reason for this is that when carbohydrate is eaten by itself, it is absorbed very quickly, which can change our hormone levels and make us hungry more quickly. Eating small amounts of protein and healthy fats with carbohydrate foods makes us feel fuller for longer, reduces overall portion size and reduces the meal's overall glycaemic index.

Many people combine nutrients in their dinner meals, some combine them with their lunch meals; however, many do not combine nutrients at breakfast and particularly when eating snacks. The nutrient that is often neglected is protein. Eating small amounts of protein throughout the day has the benefit of providing even energy throughout the day, reducing sugar cravings, moderating blood sugar levels and controlling hunger.

Breakfast and snack ideas

For optimum protein and carbohydrate combining, it is best when one serve of protein food is combined with no more than two serves of carbohydrate. We will guide you through some breakfast and snack ideas.

Breakfast

Try the following breakfast options:

- poached eggs, spinach and mushrooms on a nine-grain English muffin
- low-fat cottage cheese, capsicum, onions and smoked salmon on toast
- high fibre cereal with nuts and low-fat milk
- avocado, tomato and lean ham on wholegrain toast
- porridge with berries and protein powder.

Snacks

Try the following snack ideas:

- yoghurt
- fruit and nuts

- wholemeal or rye crackers with small amount of cheese, tomato and onion
- multigrain crackers with tinned tuna or salmon
- mini quiches without the pastry
- vegetable sticks with hummus or babaganoush.

Protein foods

One serve of protein (approximately 15 grams) equals:

- two eggs
- 75 grams (raw weight) meat (50 grams cooked)
- 75 grams (raw weight) chicken (50 grams cooked)
- 90 grams (raw weight) fish (75 grams cooked)
- 60 grams of nuts
- one small tin of tuna
- 50 grams of cheese
- 100 grams of tofu
- 1½ tablespoons of protein powder (80 per cent protein).

Carbohydrate foods

One serve of carbohydrate (approx 20 grams) equals:

- two slices of bread (thin and small)
- one medium potato
- half a cup of cooked rice
- three-quarters of a cup of cooked pasta
- one English muffin
- half a cup of starchy veggies
- 1 medium-sized serve of fruit
- 100 grams of hokkein noodles.

Proteins and carbohydrates

Combining proteins and carbohydrates is easy, while some foods naturally contain both carbohydrate and protein, for example, milk and yoghurt, as well as legumes and lentils. But be sure to eat these without added sugar or extra creamy yoghurt!

You should aim for an equal ratio of one carbohydrate serve to one protein serve. At the most, there should be one carbohydrate serve to half a protein serve.

Half a serve of protein and one serve of carbohydrate equals:

- 30 grams of nuts and one serve of fruit
- one egg and one English muffin
- 75 grams of meat and one cup of cooked rice
- 200 grams of yoghurt
- 250 millilitres of milk
- 200 grams of kidney beans, chickpeas or lentils.

Takeaway tips

- Eat protein foods with carbohydrate foods.
- Don't be enticed by low-fat, high carbohydrate snacks containing no protein.
- Portion control snacks, such as nuts, so you don't overeat.
- Reduce your carbohydrate content in meals by replacing with non-starchy vegetables.
- Remember that familiar foods are habits, and there doesn't need to be rules about what you should eat at certain times, such as for breakfast.
- Analyse your diet to see if you need to change the combinations of your meals.

Chapter 20

FEEL FREE TO HAVE THREE

We are often told that if we want to lose weight, we need to eat regularly and replace our traditional three square meals a day with six or more smaller meals a day. Controlled research has found that people who eat more often are able to lose more weight than those who eat only three meals a day. However, the difference is relatively small for many. For some people, particularly those who are emotional eaters or find it hard to keep full, changing to this eating pattern could in fact be disastrous.

In our clinic we have found that when some people increase the number of meals they have, they tend to eat a lot more throughout the day, which causes them to put on weight rather than lose it. This has also been shown in a Queensland study, which found that whether people ate three meals or six smaller meals throughout the day, weight loss is very similar. It is the overall intake that counts, not the number of times you eat. In saying this, in the Good Enough Diet we encourage you to eat three times per day at a minimum. If you eat any more than this, your meals should be smaller and your snacks healthy.

When less is less

Ben Robertson, a corporate lawyer, had let his health go for long enough. He was unfit and overweight, and at only 40 years of age was diagnosed with type 2 diabetes. Throughout school and university Ben was the perfect picture of health. He was always *big* and even scored the nickname 'Big Ben', but his size was due to pure muscle. He played representative rugby, and spent his time between parties and studying at the gym. When he started his articles year, things changed. He wasn't close to a gym and frankly didn't have the time to get to one. He was tired, so he would often sleep in, resulting in skipping breakfast and not eating until he picked up his morning latte and muffin from the coffee cart at work. He would eat when his secretary brought him some food and during meetings when there were snacks available. Ben was a single man, so he took care of his dinner meals by eating at the restaurant close to work or ordering in takeaway.

One thing that all of Big Ben's mates will tell you is that he could put it away. Whether he was eating with friends or family, at restaurants or at home, Ben was a big eater. It took him a long while to feel full and he would often gaze at everyone else's plates like a seagull ready to swoop when food was pushed to the side.

When Ben was diagnosed with type 2 diabetes, he realised that he had to make some lifestyle changes, so he started to look at his diet. His doctor told him to begin with eating six small meals per day to kickstart his metabolism before his appointment with us scheduled for two weeks later. His doctor also told him to eat breakfast every day.

When Ben came in to see us, his previous two weeks had been dreadful. He was trying to stick with his doctor's suggestions, but he had found that he'd actually increased weight. 'Maybe there is something wrong with my metabolism', said Ben. Together we looked at his diet and found the problem. Eating regularly was not going to work for Ben. He is the type of person who finds eating small amounts difficult, and when he is presented with food too often, he ends up spending most of the day thinking about food. Ben had become obsessed with eating and the more he thought about food, the more he wanted to eat.

He was now eating a healthy breakfast—a small tin of baked beans on wholegrain toast, or an omelette made in an omelette maker with wholegrain toast. He would tell us that during the morning at work, despite having just eaten, he still found himself wanting a muffin with his coffee, but had so far managed to resist it. His secretary would bring him the best option instead from the coffee cart—raisin toast.

For lunch he was now taking a proper break and eating at the restaurant he previously only frequented for dinner. Interestingly, he found that this break actually made him more productive later in the afternoon, rather than considering lunch a waste of thirty minutes that he used to think it was. It also gave him the opportunity to catch up with his co-workers, such as his secretary, one of the other partners in the firm or a junior solicitor he was mentoring, or a client.

For afternoon tea his secretary would organise a serve of fruit and a snack bar or a healthy slice. Dinner was still at the restaurant, and he was even considering buying shares in the place, since he figured he was helping out so much with the cashflow. When he got home at night he would have his second piece of fruit and something like yoghurt or a couple of healthy biscuits to ensure he ate his six meals for the day.

Despite eating all day, Ben told us that he never felt full and could always fit in something else to eat. He complained that this eating pattern was making his whole day about food. If he wasn't eating it, he was thinking about it. This was affecting his concentration at work, but at least he thought the short-term sacrifice was going to be worth it when he next jumped on the scales.

The next time Ben jumped on the scales was at our office. Although they were different scales from the ones he was used to, the 4 kilogram increase couldn't be explained by just that. Ben was not happy.

When less is less (cont'd)

What was happening to Ben was something we saw too often in our clinics—people who want to lose weight being told they need to eat more regularly to lose weight. You see, when two people eat the same amount of food but one person spreads it out over the day and the other person eats it in three meals, the person who eats more regularly will lose more weight. However, this difference is very slight, and when we don't have someone controlling what we eat, this advice could actually make us put on weight.

Some people are great at self-regulating, and if they have an additional couple of snacks per day, they reduce their meal portions accordingly. For others, the extra snacks have no effect on the portion sizes of their meals, so they end up eating more kilojoules throughout the day than they would if they had only eaten three meals with no snacks.

For Ben, this was him to a tee. He would eat his snacks, but this would rarely affect his meal portions later in the day.

To assist Ben we spoke about all of the strategies in this book to help him lose weight, but the main one was to only eat three times per day. We even gave him the times in which he was allowed to eat, and gave him a two-hour window in which he could eat his breakfast, lunch and dinner. This allowed him to contain eating to these periods, and keep his mind away from food at every other time. Ben was able to organise his day around his meal times, and we even implemented some strategies for some delicious home-cooked meals, which are discussed in chapter 22. If Ben had important meetings to attend or had to go to court over lunch or dinnertime, the plan allowed some flexibility and offered quick solutions for such times, or a meal could be shifted to work with his schedule.

Quickly, Ben's food and kilojoule intake were lower. His blood sugar levels started to stabilise, and his energy increased so he felt more motivated. Soon, without too much angst, Ben's weight dropped and still continues to fall today. Now he walks to court, cooks some meals at home and orders healthy options at his local restaurant.

Takeaway tips

- Determine whether you are an overeater or someone who finds it hard to keep full.
- Determine whether you eat more when you eat five or six meals per day.
- Eat breakfast daily — within three hours of waking.
- Define three to four meal times and give yourself a one- to two-hour time slot in which to eat them, as if you were back at school.

Chapter 21

A FAST GAME'S A GOOD GAME

Time for a quick little physiology lesson! The main way your body produces energy is through the breakdown of fat and carbohydrate (there are other sources of energy but their contribution is very small so let's not go there). The percentage of fat and carbohydrate we use for energy can vary greatly since different fuels are utilised depending on what is happening to your body. In particular, as we increase the intensity of our exercise, the percentage of fat we burn decreases. In other words, the harder we exercise the more we rely on carbohydrate as an energy source.

Following this realisation, the 'fat burning zone' was born. The fat burning zone said that to lose body fat you must exercise at a low intensity. For example, to maximise fat loss we were told to walk rather than run. The fallout of this message is that people started exercising at a slow pace. In fact, many pieces of cardio equipment are plastered with a fat burning zone diagram, complete with clear barriers, indicating the range of intensity you must exercise within to lose the most amount of body fat.

The fat burning zone

The fat burning zone is based on the intensity of the exercise you are doing. This intensity can be calculated a number of ways but the most common way is to base it upon the percentage of your maximum heart rate. Maximum heart rate is worked out by subtracting your age from the number 220. Therefore, if you are 40 years of age, your maximum heart rate is 220 – 40 = 180 beats per minute. If you are 60 years old, it will be 160 beats per minute.

The fat burning zone says that you shouldn't exercise at a level above 65 per cent of your maximum heart rate, as exercising below this burns the maximum percentage of fat. For a 40 year old this means that you can't go above 117 beats per minute. For a 60 year old you can't go above 104 beats per minute. The problem is that to stay under these heart rates you are barely able to move. If you are 60 years old and walking on a treadmill at any decent pace, your heart rate will climb to over 100 beats per minute. However, this belief was held for a number of years and exercise prescription revolved around it. Also, it became very popular because it told people not to exert themselves too much while they exercised. Basically, we gave people a licence to bludge and they embraced it with open arms.

But the whole fat burning zone theory falls down because it doesn't take into account the total amount of energy burnt during the exercise period.

Consider this — if you are exercising at a low intensity (say 50 per cent of your maximum heart rate for 30 minutes), the percentage of fat you burn may be about 40 per cent and the percentage of carbohydrate is 60 per cent. However, you only burn 750 kilojoules of energy in total. Compare that with exercising at a high intensity for 30 minutes (say 70 per cent of your maximum heart rate), where you use 80 per cent of carbohydrates and 20 per cent of fat. However, during your workout you burn 1850 kilojoules of energy. Twenty per cent of 1850 kilojoules (370 kilojoules) is more than 40 per cent of 750 kilojoules (300 kilojoules). Even though the percentage of fat you burn is less overall, the total amount of fat you use up is greater when exercising at a high intensity. Keep in mind that this doesn't include the increase in energy burnt post exercise due to an elevation in metabolism that higher intensity exercise also brings.

It's not hard to convince clients about the merits of this theory. Think about it: have you ever seen an overweight sprinter or gymnast?

They train at incredibly high intensities, yet remain very lean. For even more proof that this argument has merit check the exercise guidelines in chapter 10 which reveal that the amount of exercise necessary for good health and weight loss is reduced dramatically when you exercise vigorously.

Death by treadmill

Dianne is a 62-year-old professional woman who was diagnosed with type 2 diabetes two years ago. During this time she has worked hard on becoming more active and improving her diet. Due to her efforts she has dramatically improved her health and diabetes management. However, during this period she only lost 2 kilograms of body weight. When she came to us we discussed the type of exercise she was doing and found that she walked for one hour a day on the treadmill.

Early on she had been told about the fat burning zone and in order to stay in the target heart rate zone she could only walk at 4.5 kilometres per hour. When we watched Dianne do this she was basically ambling along. We very quickly cut her walking time down to 30 minutes and increased her speed, with intervals thrown in. At the end of the 30 minutes we also added 15 minutes of resistance training. With this new format, Dianne's heart rate ranged from 75 per cent to 85 per cent of her maximum heart rate, far above the fat burning zone.

Within a month Dianne's body weight started to drop and her body shape began to change. Over the next six months she lost 9 kilograms of body weight. Why? Because she was now exercising beyond the fat burning zone. The added bonus of her new workout was that it was shorter and more interesting. Dianne had found the one-hour walk on the treadmill mindnumbingly boring. In contrast she loved the resistance training exercises, as she felt her muscles becoming more toned, and the variety of walking in intervals also kept her interested.

There are two main messages that we can take from this:

1. There is no magical exercise intensity that will melt away your fat — don't get too caught up on working in a certain zone.
2. Higher intensity exercise will help you lose more body fat, as well as get you fitter and healthier.

How you use this practically is the most important issue here. When it comes to weight loss, exercise as hard as you can manage. To be good enough this doesn't mean you have to exhaust yourself every time you work out, just get out of cruise mode. Also remember that your exercise needs to be relative to your fitness level. If you are unfit, high intensity for you may be a brisk walk; however, if you are moderately active, high intensity might be a jog. Aim to continually but gradually increase the intensity of the exercise you do.

Increasing your intensity

We will now provide some examples for how to increase your exercise intensity if your chosen exercise is walking, followed by some tips for resistance training.

In the gym on a treadmill

An obvious way to increase the intensity if you are walking on a treadmill is to break into a jog at different points during your walk. However, if you don't enjoy running, the challenge is that you can only walk so fast. If you get to the point where you can no longer increase your walking speed, the next step is to increase the elevation of the treadmill. The higher you make the elevation, the greater the intensity will be.

Walking outdoors

As with walking on a treadmill, the obvious choice to increase the intensity if you are walking outdoors is to throw in some jogging. An even better option would be to find a walking route with hills to increase your intensity further. To take your walking intensity to a new level, incorporate some stairs in your workout. Find a set of stairs and climb them at different points during your walk. You don't just have to climb them once. You can use the walk back down the stairs for your rest and repeat this over again and again.

Resistance training

When it comes to resistance training there are three ways to increase your intensity:

1   Increase the weight that you lift.
2   Increase how many times you lift the weight.
3   Reduce the rest time between exercises.

As you can see, increasing the intensity of your exercise will not only improve your health, it will also get you faster weight loss results.

How to work out your exercise intensity

There are many ways to work out your exercise intensity but by far the simplest is the 'talk test' as shown in table 21.1. It involves seeing how well you can talk while exercising. If you are a little short of breath when you exercise but you find it easy to have a conversation, you are exercising at a *low intensity*. If you can still talk but it is much harder to make complete sentences, you are reaching *medium intensity*. If you find it difficult to answer in anything more than a few words, it's likely that you are working at a *high intensity*.

Table 21.1: the talk test

Talk test	Intensity
Can hold conversation easily	Low
Can hold conversation	Medium
Unable to talk	High

Takeaway tips

- Exercise as hard as you can — medium to high intensity.
- Look at your current exercise program and work out a plan to increase the intensity, whether that means introducing intervals, increasing the overall speed of your walk or run, including hills or walking up stairs, or increasing how much you lift if you are resistance training.
- When increasing intensity do it gradually as you don't want to be too sore the next day and unable to exercise, or become injured.

Part V GOOD ENOUGH IN REAL LIFE

Chapter 22

HEALTH IN A HURRY

When you think about 'health in a hurry', you may consider it as much of an oxymoron as healthy fast food. The truth is, that with a bit of understanding, both can be suitable realities in your weight loss journey.

Working long hours is common for many of us, along with busy families and all of the accompanying responsibilities. On top of this, we have extracurricular activities that we try to fit in, from artistic pursuits to sports to catching up with friends. Life couldn't be more full, so the last thing you want to think about is cooking yourself a healthy meal when you get home. For many of us, the demands of home life can be a bigger stress than the dread of starting a busy work day.

Today there are loads of health in a hurry solutions that can be incorporated into your weight loss routine to make life easier for you. You only have the ability to maintain a certain level of mental and physical energy, so with options such as home-delivered meals, quick dinners, online shopping, eating out and frozen dinners, you can free up more energy for the really important things.

Eating out

City living and working in the corporate world can seem like the ultimate lifestyle/career move, but they can also be disastrous for your health, as more often than not your work will require you to eat out at restaurants and your lifestyle demands will mean that takeaway is relied upon more often than traditionally seen as healthy.

Challenges of a high flyer

Greg Butler is the principal certified accountant at a busy accounting firm in the city. As well as his accounting work, he sits on a number of boards, which mean hours and hours of commuting in planes and time spent in meetings. Greg was too busy to come to our office, so we went to him. We knew how busy he was, and that a perfect, well-prepared diet may not be achievable. But Greg did need to lose weight—at 126 kilograms his weight was expanding as quickly as his career success. We had to do something. 'I want to lose weight, but my work comes first, and any spare time I have I want to share with my kids', he shared with us. 'I can't be sitting there chewing on rabbit food or looking like I'm eating from a bird feeder while everyone else is eating takeaway or pastries.'

For many of us, travelling and eating out is a treat, so we treat ourselves with extra courses, richer meals and bigger portions. However, when you travel twice a week, wait around for flights in airport lounges with all the trimmings, and dine in restaurants more regularly than you eat at home, you can't afford to eat like this—and Greg certainly was no exception. Lucky for us, most of Greg's work was based in familiar places, and was planned out months in advance. His executive assistant, Tanya, is super efficient. When Greg travels he not only has everything in his iPhone synchronised with his computer diary, but Tanya prepares a clear document file that includes copies of every piece of information he might need, from printouts of his flights and accommodation to emails or company information required for his meetings. She told us, 'Greg's so busy when he travels. I need to make sure he can find everything

> easily when he needs it, and when he travels straight from one meeting to the next he needs to be able to switch quickly. One thing I haven't mastered is his food — he just grabs whatever's available and when he's hungry, as you can imagine, he doesn't always make the best choices'.
>
> With Tanya's help, we went to work. We examined every aspect of Greg's schedule, the airport lounges he would be waiting in, the flights he would be taking, the meetings he would be attending, the accommodation he was using and the restaurants/events that he would be attending.
>
> It is amazing that when you focus on healthy eating and exercise, there is always a solution available. Even when your only options are fast-food restaurants, there will always be a healthy choice on the menu. With the pre-planning done, Greg was able to work in any situation and have healthy foods available whenever he needed them. Hotel and restaurant staff are extremely accommodating when it comes to creating special meals, and even when advising caterers of special events of Greg's dietary requirements, we have never had a problem organising a healthy option for him.

Greg's story will be familiar for many of us who work extra-long hours and compromise our health and diet for the demands of our career and family responsibilities. In chapter 23 we discuss travelling success, but let's first look at how we can eat out at restaurants and order from takeaway and fast-food outlets and still lose weight.

Healthy eating out

The closer *all* of your meals can be to the healthy meals you can prepare at home, the healthier they will be, and the healthier *you* will be. This applies to all types of foods and portions.

The main ingredients

It's a simple rule and discussed often throughout this book: ensure that half of your plate is made up of non-starchy vegetables. It's the most effective way to reduce the kilojoule content of your meal, increase your nutrient and fibre intake, and help you to feel full. Regardless of how unhealthy your meal is, it is only half as bad if you only eat half of it. If you would usually eat a whole pizza, share it, along with a shared green salad. If you would usually eat a pasta meal, share it and share a side of steamed vegetables, too. You can always ask the chef to make you half-size meals if you're eating by yourself. Be warned, waiters will look at you strangely, but after you have done it a few times the awkwardness will fade, and you will be happy to be in control of your own meals. While you are already being a nuisance, make sure you ask for extra non-starchy vegetables, cooked without oil or butter, and your dressing to be placed on the side.

After you have ensured you have the main thing (vegetables) down, the next step is to ensure the protein you are eating is lean. Fish is one food that many Australians don't eat enough of, so if you can order baked or grilled fish as your first option, you are doing really well. Chicken should have the skin removed, and other cuts of meat should have the visible fat removed. It is best to cut all fat off any meats as soon as you get your meal to reduce the urge to eat it. Eating deep-fried meats and fish is an easy way to add on the kilos, so always request that your meats are uncoated and not fried. Yes, this means limited battered and crumbed options.

Now for the fibre content of your meal. It is a rare treat for the health conscious, but hopefully restaurants will start to include more wholegrain, wholemeal and brown options to help us reach our daily fibre needs and keep our blood sugar levels at a more even level.

The final point on your checklist when eating out is to ensure that dishes don't contain any fatty or sugary condiments, often hidden in sauces or mixes. Cream and butter are common ingredients in egg dishes, curries and sauces. If in doubt, ask, or go for safer options, such as tomato-based sauces and vinegar-based dressings, and always ask for sauces and dressings to be served on the side.

Hidden dangers

When eating out, the meals that are the most obvious unhealthy choices are not really problems for our clients who are trying to lose weight. Instead the problem is with the *salads* and *low-fat* options that people think are the healthiest things to eat on the menu. We are still amazed at the number of people who order Caesar salads when they are trying to be good. Let's look at this rationally. Throughout this book we have encouraged you to eat non-starchy vegetables with each of your meals (see chapter 3). When you look at the ingredients in a Caesar salad, you are right in noticing that cos lettuce is a non-starchy vegetable, but when you consider the bacon, egg, parmesan cheese, croutons (usually deep-fried) and anchovies... these are not non-starchy vegetables. Add the fattening creamy dressing and this *salad* contains the same amount of kilojoules as a hamburger and French fries. A rice salad is a rice dish, not a salad. A potato salad is a potato dish, not a salad. A pasta salad is a pasta dish, not a salad. A salad contains non-starchy vegetables. Some additions, including protein options such as cheese, nuts or meats, are okay, as long as most of the salad contains non-starchy vegetables.

Choosing healthy food is just one part of the eating-out maze. Sadly, value is often associated with the size of meals and therefore restaurants serve bigger meals than you may eat at home. These oversized portions can easily add weight to your waistline as it's all too easy to overeat, even if the food is healthy. 'There is always that urge to eat everything on your plate', says Greg, 'but I have been taught to always push what I will eat to the side and only eat that amount. I also don't eat the breads, starters or dessert. Not easy... but extremely important'. If Greg has a fridge in his room, when he gets his meal he often asks for a takeaway container. Before he starts his meal, he portions what he needs and packs away the remaining amount, which then makes for a great breakfast or lunch the following day.

Tips for healthy eating out

If you're like Greg and struggle to eat healthily when you go out for a meal, take a look at the following handy tips:

- Aim for half your meal to contain non-starchy vegetables or salads.
- Where possible choose brown or wholemeal rice, pasta or noodles.
- Choose meat, chicken and fish that is uncoated and not deep-fried.
- Request that your meal is cooked in less oil or butter.
- Choose tomato- or vinegar-based sauces and dressings over creamy, oily or buttery sauces.

- If you want to treat yourself when you eat out, reserve it for special occasions, which would match a regular person's lifestyle.
- Never assume anything. Always ask about the ingredients in your meals, and don't always trust 'healthy' symbols.
- Ask for dressings and sauces to be served on the side.
- Choose smaller portions.
- If possible, check out the restaurant menu beforehand, so you are not tempted by the look or smell of the meals being served around you.
- If you are travelling, find out where healthy restaurants or takeaways are located in relation to your workplace or hotel.
- If you are attending conferences where food is provided, don't be afraid to ask for a healthier meal.

Healthy fast food

So, what if you have left dinner to the last minute? What if you have nothing planned? What if there is nothing healthy open? What if the war on your weight is a barrier of fast-food chains that you have to navigate your way through?

Luckily, fast-food chains are starting to offer lots of healthier options. And many places now display the kilojoule content of their meals and highlight their healthy choices.

But you can't always trust the healthier choices highlighted by a fast-food chain. An item may be low in fat, but the portion size will make it an unhealthy option. Or it may be low in kilojoules, but when accompanied with a soft drink and large fries, it won't be a better choice.

Like all areas of your diet, when eating fast food the main issue is to get some non-starchy vegetables in your meal, and the more the better. And the better you will be doing if you also reduce the amount of deep-fried food you order, or food laden with unhealthy additions such as butter, cream, sour cream, oily dressings or cheese.

Some options, like Asian dishes, may seem to have all the attributes of a healthy meal, but can be cooked in what seems like a barrel of oil. If your meal will be cooked fresh, ask for more vegetables and less oil.

If it will be served from a bain-marie, you can usually see if there is oil rising to the top of the dish and you can choose a better option.

If you really have no choice but to eat something unhealthy, see what you can do to make it healthier. Ask for no butter, mayonnaise or other creamy sauces to be served with your meal, and request an additional salad or vegetables if possible.

Health in a hurry in action

Just walking in to see Tony Lye, a fit and healthy looking 60-year-old man, makes my eyes light up. Tony Lye is a legend in the insurance world. He is a pioneer who shaped the way insurance is carried out in Australia. Tony is one of those people who is loved wherever he goes due to his zest for life and infectious enthusiasm. He has energy to burn, and he's successful and happy. He seems to be on top of everything — his career, his family and his weight... But it hasn't always been this way.

Like many of our clients, Tony has been super successful in his career and family life, but despite being confident and competent in every other area of his life, he couldn't get on top of his weight. Tony has battled this for his entire life, with a history of losing weight (sometimes up to 30 kilograms) using different diets but always putting it back on — unfortunately with interest.

At his heaviest Tony was 165 kilograms. With high cholesterol and narrowing of the blood vessels that kept his heart ticking, he was a heart attack waiting to happen. And while his heart was still pumping, his lungs were in trouble. Tony also had severe sleep apnoea, a condition that stops sufferers from breathing in their sleep and requires the wearing of a special breathing mask at night.

For 30 years Tony had been a competitive rugby player, so the exercise component of our weight loss program didn't concern him too much. In fact, he was excited about getting back into exercise. The real stumbling block for Tony was his diet. He had been on every diet imaginable but found that all of the traditional diet approaches interfered with his career and family life.

Health in a hurry in action (cont'd)

Although it would have been preferable for Tony to make his own meals and use fresh ingredients daily, Tony couldn't commit to this type of diet—as soon as a busy day came up his good work would quickly come undone. We discussed the option of having the weight management company Lite n' Easy deliver portion-controlled meals to his home. First of all we identified Tony's requirements and even tried the meals ourselves to ensure they were suitable. Tony found this more than acceptable. He liked the food. It was inexpensive. It was delivered to his door. Best of all, Tony didn't have to think about what he ate; it was all done for him. It was cooked, prepared, and even labelled with the day and meal that it should be eaten.

Today Tony is down to 98 kilograms. He is exercising daily and loving it. His sleep apnoea and heart health have improved dramatically and he is fitter than he ever thought possible.

A few months ago Tony's weight loss started to slow. Rather than losing 1 kilogram a week he was losing around 1 kilogram every three weeks. We thought it was due to his body getting closer to his goal weight of 90 kilograms. Then a month later Tony's work schedule exploded and he was to travel for 29 days out of the month. We were all very concerned about the fact that Tony's hard work would all come undone, since he wouldn't have access to his home-delivered meals and he couldn't perform his regular exercise routine. In preparation for this time we worked with Tony on implementing the dining out strategies discussed throughout this book. Fast forward to the time of writing and Tony has come out the other side of his travel month from hell, 5 kilograms lighter. His weight loss actually accelerated throughout this period, instead of stalling or going backwards.

Home-delivered meals

The secret to Tony's success is that he stuck to his plan and was consistent. His weight loss strategy fitted in with his work and lifestyle, but an essential element to his success was the convenience and practicality of home-delivered meals.

Some of our clients have decided to take a similar road to Tony, with all meals being home-delivered. However, many have found that they order just a few home-delivered meals to have on hand in case something comes up and preparing a meal isn't an option.

Tony is lucky—he is working with a team that helps him choose his food, but also gives him support to eat similarly when he does have time to cook for himself. 'I get the advice from my team on what to order, but I feel like I learn from the program—particularly with portion sizes. I find the protein recommended is smaller than I was used to, and there are a lot more vegetables than I ever ate before. I now know what a balanced meal should look like.'

Tony's story is a perfect example of when near enough is more than good enough to lose weight. You may not want to eat frozen and pre-prepared meals all the time, but if you keep some in the freezer at work or at home they might come in handy when something unexpected pops up.

Home-delivered meal options

We recommend the following home-delivered meal services:

- Lite n' Easy <www.liteneasy.com.au>
- Tender Loving Cuisine <www.tlc.org.au/index.jsp>
- Jenny Craig <www.jennydirect.com.au>.

Quick dinners

Sometimes work and life don't go as planned. This means that organised meals can fall by the wayside. You might have done everything perfectly—organised your weekly meal plan and shopping list, and even thawed your meat, but in the end time gets away and you just want something quickly.

They may not be *MasterChef* quality, but quick and easy meals can be perfectly healthy and a great option for when time is scarce or you haven't been able to shop. Always make sure you have some emergency supplies available in case something goes wrong and you still want to eat healthily and at home.

Really, quick and easy cooking is a no-brainer. We have included a few meals ideas to show you how simply it can be done, but the options will only be restricted by your imagination and what is in your pantry.

- Always ensure you have some non-starchy vegetables available. Stocking a wide range of frozen and tinned vegetables can be a great back up, or if you know you'll eat them within a few days, pre-chopped salads are also very handy.

- Protein sources such as lean meats, chicken or fish can be easily frozen until you want to use them. You can also buy meats that are diced or sliced so they are ready to use. Vegetarian options such as tofu and tempeh take less time to cook, as do eggs, and will last in the fridge a lot longer than meat. For a super simple option, tinned fish like salmon and even tinned chicken are great options to always keep in your pantry.

- If you have exercised in the afternoon, you will need to eat carbohydrates with your dinner as well. Practically no preparation is needed to eat a slice of heavy-grained, low glycaemic index (GI) bread; however, even rice can be cooked in less time than it will take you to have a shower. Rice cookers make it easy to serve carbohydrates in a hurry, but quicker options are now available with two-minute microwavable pastas and rice. Where possible choose higher fibre options, such as brown rice, wholegrain pasta or multigrain bread, and always have these handy in your pantry.

If you keep your pantry and freezer properly stocked, you should never have to resort to dialling for a curry in a hurry again and blowing your diet! Here's a suggested checklist of what to keep stocked at home so the cupboard is never bare and your weight management is that little bit easier...

In the pantry:

- *Proteins.* Tins of fish; tinned chicken breast; tins of beans and legumes (kidney beans, chickpeas, four bean mix).

- *Carbohydrates.* Quick cook brown or basmati rice; brown rice or udon noodles; wholemeal pasta; thin multigrain wrap or lavash bread; tinned corn.

- *Vegetables.* Tinned tomatoes.

In the fridge:

- *Proteins.* Eggs; meat to cook within a few days; fish to cook within a few days; hard tofu.
- *Vegetables.* Non-starchy vegetables and salad; pre-cut vegetables and salads (you can buy them cut, or you can do this yourself).
- *Meals.* Leftovers or cooked meals that can be eaten within 72 hours.

In the freezer:

- *Proteins.* Meat, chicken or fish that you portion yourself or buy pre-portioned.
- *Vegetables.* Frozen vegetables, including beans, broccoli, cauliflower, brussels sprouts, spinach and steam-fresh mixed vegetable pouches.
- *Meals.* Frozen meals either pre-purchased or made from leftovers.

Frozen dinners

The ultimate easy meal is one that's prepared ready to go just after you arrive home. Frozen leftovers are a simple option. Whenever you prepare a meal, make enough so that you can create an additional meal and eat this when you don't have time or don't feel like cooking.

Following are some helpful guidelines if you are freezing your own meals:

- Freeze meals within two hours of cooking them.
- Don't refrigerate and freeze, or thaw and refreeze.
- Freeze meals in individual portions.
- Always freeze your meals in containers or ziplock bags.
- Ensure that your portions are the same size as your normal dinner. You can do this by transferring the portion onto a plate and then into a container.
- Meals with lots of sauce, such as pasta sauces, curries or stews, will freeze better than dry meals.

- It may be easier to freeze sauces separately from the dish that they will be eaten with. For example, pasta sauces can be frozen separately to pasta.
- Some vegetables don't freeze as well as others in meals. Dicing vegetables like mushrooms and onions will ensure they reheat well and taste as good as they would in a freshly cooked meal.
- Meals should be eaten within two months of freezing.

If you don't have leftovers available, another option is to stock commercially prepared frozen dinners. With advances in food technology, there are now better tasting meals than ever before, and there is a variety of healthy choices, too.

The rules to follow when eating frozen dinners are the same as when eating quick and easy dinners and when eating out. Look for lots of veggies — and if the meal doesn't contain enough, which is common, add some extra frozen veggies or a salad. You'll find that the portions are usually pretty small, but enough for a meal.

What to look for in a commercial frozen dinner

Following are some things to look out for in a commercial frozen dinner:

- If you are trying to lose weight, the energy per meal should be between 1500 kilojoules and 2000 kilojoules.
- Make sure protein makes up at least 12 grams per meal.
- Choose high fibre and low GI meals.
- Choose varieties that you enjoy.

Online shopping

Having 20 minutes a day to cook a meal is one thing, but having the time to shop is another. You go to the supermarket full of hope and promise, yet end up wandering aimlessly through the aisles wishing that a meal would leap out and say 'Here I am. Cook me'.

However, a beacon of hope is out there — it's called online shopping. Truly a gift from the heavens! You are able to select your groceries in the comfort of your own home, and plan what you will cook simultaneously. The next day, your shopping magically appears in your kitchen!

Besides the convenience of getting only what you want and not buying extras due to the lure of advertising and sales items in the supermarket, brand positioning or your level of hunger, online shopping also means no more calf injuries from kids hitting you with a trolley, no more tantrums in public (I mean you, not the kids) and no more death stares when you try to sneak 15 items through the 12 items or less checkout.

Technology is often seen as a detriment to your health, but the truth is that you can't beat it. So why not use it to make you healthier? The seven minutes it takes you to purchase your groceries online as opposed to the two hours it takes going to the local supermarket is worth the price of admission all by itself.

What would you rather do, spend time relaxing or push a trolley? An even better option is to dedicate the time you save from shopping to exercising with a friend or a work colleague.

Online shopping options

Here are the main players in the market:

- Coles <www.colesonline.com.au>
    - Delivery is nationwide, day or night, so you can set up your order to suit your time schedule.
    - Minimum order is $30.
    - Delivery charge varies from $0 to $15 depending on delivery time and location.
- Woolworths <www.homeshop.com.au>
    - An advantage is that you don't have to pay via credit card — you can pay with eftpos upon delivery.
    - Minimum order is $30.
    - Delivery charge varies from $0 to $15 depending on delivery time and location.
- Organicfood.com.au <www.organicfood.com.au>
    - Services Sydney and Melbourne.
    - Its fruit and veggies are organic and sourced from local markets. It also sells a wide range of grocery items.

- If you don't know what you want, you can order from a wide range of weekly 'organic mixed boxes', including classic and seasonal fruit and veggies, as well as essential grocery items.
- You also receive nutrition information delivered with your order, along with great recipes. This information is also available on its extensive website.

Losing weight with health in a hurry

Health in a hurry is easy to achieve, and although the options are not 100 per cent perfect, meals that the average Australian consumes are also not 100 per cent perfect.

As Greg and Tony have found, losing weight is possible without putting a massive focus on it or expending loads of time on it. You can have a healthy life, as well as one that matches your career and personal goals.

Takeaway tips

- Be healthy when you can. Do your best when you can't.
- Always include non-starchy vegetables with every meal.
- Plan your food based upon your schedule.
- Check your portions and say no to additional courses.
- Look out for the extras, like sauces, dressings and condiments.

Chapter 23

TRAVELLING SUCCESS

When you take the occasional holiday, it's fair enough to relax your healthy eating standards. However, when you are travelling regularly or you will be away for an extended period, or if you're trying to meet specific goals, you will need to be aware of what you eat when you travel.

At the airport

We often arrive at the airport in a rush. Regardless of how early we leave home or work, we have all experienced the stress of finalising last-minute details and then dealing with bumper-to-bumper traffic along the way, so most of us are already feeling ill at ease when we finally reach the airport. This can mean we forget to eat before our flight, and unless we have access to a lounge, our only options are coffee shops, newsagents and fast-food outlets.

    We will discuss the fast-food maze later in this section, but if you have limited time and your flight doesn't serve food, it is best to find something that is as close as possible to the meal that you would be eating if you weren't flying.

If you are travelling during the middle of the day and you have missed lunch, this is usually easily fixed as many airport coffee shops serve sandwiches, which can be good options. Try to choose a sandwich containing (in order of importance) some type of salad, wholegrain bread without butter or mayonnaise, and lean meat, chicken or fish. Another good option is a salad from a salad bar.

If you are hungry, but can't find a healthy meal, fruit or fruit salad is often available and a good choice. Nut bars (with lots of nuts) or muesli bars aren't the best options, but they are better than some of the baked options, such as low-fat fruit muffins or banana bread. These may seem like a good option, especially for a snack, but most contain as many kilojoules as a main meal or at least the equivalent of a couple of chocolate bars.

Airport lounges

Now that meetings are finished, your bags have been checked and you've made your way through the long security lines, the airport lounge beckons. The friendly lounge attendant greets you at the door and it's the first time you've had all day to read the newspaper. You are relaxed.

What better way to pass the time than with a couple of glasses of your favourite red and a few nibbles courtesy of the airline. What better way to put on a few extra kilos over the year. Wine, beer and spirits are not water. They contain kilojoules, and as you read in chapter 7, they are not insignificant.

And as you read in chapter 4, all of the small savoury bites and sweet delights will tempt you to eat more than you planned to and smorgasbord syndrome will take over.

Surviving airport lounges

Remember when you were a child and you would eat fish and chips on the beach? If you were anything like us, your favourite thing was to throw a chip into a huge flock of seagulls and watch them go nuts over it. A similar thing happens in airport lounges when a lounge attendant brings out the meat pies. All of a sudden sophisticated businesspeople in their smart suits turn into human seagulls and literally trample each other to get to the food.

On the contrary, it is possible to survive airport lounges. Firstly, if you are a regular traveller, stay away from the alcohol. You are just drinking empty kilojoules, meaning actual kilojoules but no beneficial nutrients. If you do have a drink, stick to one of the better choices — like a small glass of wine, a light beer, or a spirit with soda (see chapter 7 for more options).

Airport lounges are quite large, and although there are not always seats available where you want to sit, try to find one away from the food and drinks so they are out of sight. When you can see food, particularly moreish food like lollies or savoury nibbles, you will eat more of them even if you don't intend to.

If you are in an airport lounge during a meal time, choose a healthy option. I have never been to an airport lounge that didn't have fruit and salad available. Wholegrain bread and lean proteins, like ham or tuna, are also regularly available. If only snack food is being served, even a little bit does matter, so it's best to stay away. Determine whether you are really hungry, as you will usually be able to go without until your flight.

Travel trouble

When you fly, particularly on long flights, to different time zones or during strange hours of the day, keeping on top of your nutrition and hydration can make all the difference to your weight and, of course, your energy levels when you arrive at your destination. Often we are required to jump off the flight and straight into a meeting, and since the locals attending will be on their game, we need to be, too.

Flying can also have dreadful effects on your bowels if you travel regularly. By ensuring when you're at home that you drink plenty of water and fluids — about 1.8 litres to 2 litres daily — eat lots of fibre (see chapter 3) and also take probiotic drinks such as Yakult, which contain good bacteria, you will help keep your bowels working well throughout your travelling life.

Travelling time

When you are on the flight, it is best to stick to your usual meal routine, rather than eating everything you will be served. Airlines usually feed you every three to five hours, which is fine when you're busy and walking around but too much when you are doing nothing but sitting down.

If you are in business or first class on international flights, it is possible to specify when you would like to eat. Although airlines say they offer this service, from experience we're not sure that they fully embrace this yet; however, if you are a regular traveller, it is important that you take up this option. So what do you eat and when?

Firstly, you need to make a choice and stick to it from the moment you arrive at the airport. Will you be eating according to your usual time, or eating according to your location time? There is no rule as to what is best, but if you are travelling to a different time zone for less than three days, it will be easier on your body if you try to eat meals at the same time as your usual time zone if possible. It doesn't mean that the meals need to be the same type of meals, but eating at similar times will be helpful. To make this easier, you can create a travel plan, as shown in table 23.1, for your food to correspond with when you would ordinarily eat at home. For example, if you are travelling to Los Angeles, the following simple conversion can help.

Table 23.1: time zone meal travel plan

Sydney	Meal	Los Angeles	Meal
6.00 am	Breakfast	12.00 pm	Lunch
1.00 pm	Lunch	7.00 pm	Dinner
9.00 pm	Dinner	3.00 am	Breakfast

It initially seems strange, but keeping your sleeping times similar (for short trips) can also help. We don't recommend waking up early or going to sleep late when you have to work on local time, but if you only have a couple of meetings and can afford to rest when you are not busy, this is your best option.

If you are travelling for a long period (longer than a week) or you need to work a normal day, it is best to convert your meal times to your final destination's time zone as soon as you get on the plane. Again, plan this before you leave.

When we worked with Greg, the accountant from 'Challenges of a high flyer' discussed in chapter 22, we made travel plans for each of the cities he visited regularly—Auckland, Singapore, Hong Kong, Los Angeles and New York. Using time conversions, as well as details of the meals the airline served, the hotels he stayed in, and the restaurants located near his accommodation and his offices, we created a travel plan that covered each meal scenario that Greg would come across during his entire trip.

Healthy inflight meals

To make healthy eating easier during flights, many frequent flyer programs allow you to indicate meal preferences, such as a low-fat meal, a heart healthy meal or a diabetic meal. Even if you don't have a health problem, any of these options will be better than the regular ones available, and many airlines allow you to view their menus online. Since the airlines actually do respond to customer feedback, let them know that you would like healthier choices, and if it becomes a regular request, it will soon be a regular option for us all to enjoy.

Choosing the healthiest option on the flight is relatively easy, but controlling the portion sizes is another story. Although the meal itself is usually a good size, the added extras of crackers, chocolate, bread and desserts could make even a healthy meal a little too heavy. Remember, if you overeat, it becomes a waste in your body, as it would be in the bin. If you know you don't have self-control, ask the flight attendant to serve you just the side salad and main meal without the extras.

If you are on a flight where meals aren't included, there are a couple of things you can do. Don't be tempted to purchase the snacks that are always available inflight. Try to choose meals instead that meet our guidelines as discussed in chapter 3 — lots of non-starchy vegetables with lean protein and small amounts of carbohydrates. Unfortunately, some airlines just don't offer healthy choices, which can make it difficult to stick to your diet. However, many airlines allow you to bring your own food onto the flight, and armed with the information from chapter 22, you will be able to choose a great option to take with you.

Preparing for take-off

Adam, co-author of this book, normally flies business class when he travels, which fortunately always serves very healthy meal options consisting of protein and non-starchy vegetables. However, when he travels on one of the budget airlines that don't serve food, he has a strategy to avoid the junk food cart. Prior to the flight Adam will grab a salad from an airport salad bar and bring this on the flight with him. When everyone else is eating ice creams, lollies and snack bars, he is tucking into a fresh salad, allowing him to arrive at his destination with more energy and fewer kilojoules on board.

Packing your pantry

Before you start packing your pantry to bring along with you, make sure you are aware if there any restrictions on food being brought into the destination you will be travelling to. Some places forbid fresh fruit or unpackaged food, so it is important to check first. Keep in mind, though, that these foods can be eaten during your flight but will need to be discarded before you land.

However, if there are no restrictions on the food products you are bringing in, you can pack all the foods you need for your weight loss to continue while you travel, plus reduce the stress associated with trying to work out what you will eat.

Last year, Adam spent over 60 nights away from home while on speaking engagements. He is quite good when it comes to choosing healthy meals for lunch and dinner, but his biggest weakness is the breakfast buffet — the bacon and eggs seem to call out his name. But just the sight of these takes him back to his honeymoon, when he put on 7 kilograms in 10 days. So, to manage this, he always takes his own breakfast when he travels — a mix of oats, nuts, seeds and muesli — along with sliced fresh apple and milk, which he can get from most of the hotels that he stays in.

The practicalities of taking food with you needs to be managed as well, especially if the meals you are bringing need to be portioned or pre-prepared. For your travel kitchen we suggest also packing a sharp knife (you will have to check this in with your main luggage or it will be confiscated if it's in your carry-on luggage), some ziplock bags and a few paper towels.

School lunchboxes are very handy to use, especially compartmentalised ones, and can easily hold enough fresh fruit and vegetables to last three to four days. Apples, carrots, baby cucumbers, capsicum and/or broccoli make a great mix of snacks and can be put into ziplock bags and then placed in the fridge when you arrive at your destination.

Nuts are also a good snack to bring with you. You can buy them in pre-portioned packages, or take some from a larger bag and store them in small ziplock bags.

If you know you are going be busy while you travel and could skip a meal, packing some meal replacement bars or shakes may be a good option. Friends of ours — an older couple — went to Europe for a holiday for four weeks. They were worried that they wouldn't like the food (I know, who doesn't like European food?), so they filled their suitcase with meal replacement shakes. They each had two meal replacements per day (usually breakfast and lunch) and ate just one restaurant meal per day. They both came back a lot leaner, and by only eating one restaurant meal per day, they enjoyed using the extra money that they saved on shopping. We are not suggesting you go this far, but it shows how easy an alternative these meal replacements are.

Planning your travel food

Planning the food you will eat when you travel is simple with the range of technologies available to us today.

As we have discussed earlier in this book, if you are trying to lose weight it's a great help to know where the dining options are located around your accommodation, along with menus, opening times and delivery options.

Using the wisdom of crowds from social media like Twitter, Facebook, Foursquare and Yelp will also be of huge benefit to you. Asking about healthy places to eat will always generate a flurry of support and suggestions. And the great thing about social media is that you can do this ahead of time, or as compensation when you're being reactive. You never know, you might even find someone to share a meal with you.

There's really no excuse not to eat well, since most food outlets and restaurants have websites or some kind of web presence, so it will be easy to find them. Google Earth is also extremely helpful.

Tara was travelling to New York City in winter one year and was dreading the thought of having to go out in the cold to find appropriate places to eat. However, a quick scan of the neighbourhood around her hotel on Google Earth, followed by checking each of the restaurants' and takeaway food outlets' menus online, meant healthy food could be delivered easily and quickly between grocery shops. Of course, the US is known for the sizes of its meals, so often even though the meals were healthy, she did need to spread each meal over two.

The travel challenge

Travelling presents many challenges when trying to stay active. When we tell our clients that they should continue to exercise when they travel, they look at us as if we have grown another head. However, the best way to see any city is on foot — it allows you to touch, taste, smell and feel the place. Walking is especially good in cities where hiring a car is costly, and traffic and different road rules can often be confusing. For those holidays where you just sit on a bus and drive through different cities, you might as well have stayed at home and watched a DVD.

Not only can exercising on your holiday help you lose body fat or at least keep it off while you are away, it can actually add to the quality of your holiday. If you are on a skiing trip, consider finishing the day with a walk (outside or at the gym) and a few stretches. This will help reduce the soreness you will feel the next day and prevent a skiing injury.

An unfortunate drawback when you travel is that carrying all those heavy bags around can lead to both neck and back pain. A swim or a walk at the end of the day followed by some basic stretches will loosen those areas and protect you from injury or pain.

Travelling fit

Peter and Dianne are a middle-aged couple who lead a reasonably healthy lifestyle. They have always been regular exercisers (walking a couple of times per week) and have a well-balanced diet. However, both were carrying a few extra kilograms due to their hectic work schedules. When they planned a three-month trip around the world, they decided that they would use their holiday to get back down to their ideal weights. To do this they made a very clear set of five rules for their holiday:

- *Rule 1.* At each place they visited they had to do a walking tour.

- *Rule 2.* Whenever possible they would always walk rather than take a taxi (in Manhattan they set a goal to walk everywhere).

- *Rule 3.* They took a pedometer (which counts the number of steps you take) with them and any day that they didn't reach their allotted 15 000 steps they had to go for a walk until they went beyond this amount.

- *Rule 4.* No alcohol was to be consumed during the whole trip. Money saved was spent on experiences.

- *Rule 5.* In Italy they were only allowed one sweet or gelato once a day (probably the hardest rule).

How to incorporate formal exercise

It's easy to incorporate incidental exercise while you travel (exercise that serves a purpose; for example, sightseeing or walking to a museum). While incidental exercise is important, if you want to come back from your travels looking fabulous you will need to consider formal exercise too.

In order to facilitate this, book a hotel with a gym rather than a room with a view. That's right, many hotels today do have gyms. While some are flash and fabulous, others are a little on the small side. Working out in the gym is a great way to start your day and a much better way to spend your evening than watching TV in your hotel room. Don't be concerned if it doesn't have your usual machines as it's likely to have some dumbbells and at least one piece of cardiovascular equipment — a treadmill or a bike or a rower. A gym is also really useful if the weather is poor and you can't go out for a walk, or it's dark outside and you're travelling alone.

Before you go

As the Scouts say, be prepared! While there are many things you need to pack when you travel, ensuring you have the right gear can make all the difference. A pair of good walking shoes or runners, one set of clothes you can exercise in and even a pair of swimmers will allow you to swim, walk, cycle or use a gym during your travels.

And if you are feeling adventurous, you may want to investigate cycling tours — yes, these include the bike! There are some amazing cycling tours available in Europe and Asia. People who have done them say that on a bike is the only way to see a country. If you think even further outside the box, you could go on a swimming holiday in the Greek Islands, where you swim between different islands. These cater for all swimming levels and you can get on and off the boat as often as you require. What a way to see one of the most beautiful oceans on the planet!

Use available resources

Ask the concierge! It's the job of the person at your hotel desk to know the destination better than anyone. They will know where the good parks and walking tracks are located, and can point you in the right direction for a walk with a new view. Alternatively, if you want to do some formal exercise, they will be able to suggest a local gym or pool if your hotel doesn't have one, or other local activities, such as yoga, horse riding or even ice-skating!

A hotel room workout

That's right, if all else fails — the weather is dreadful and there is no gym — you can use the walls and items in your hotel room. Here are some suggestions (you will find full descriptions of the following exercises in appendix D):

- wall press against a wall or push-ups on the floor
- squats or sit to stand over a chair
- tricep dips off a chair or bed
- lunges on the spot or across the room
- the plank.

If you do resistance training, you could consider filling your backpack and wearing it while doing these exercises for extra resistance.

One of the easiest and best pieces of equipment is an exercise band. It's basically a huge rubber band that you can do just about any exercise with and it will become your own portable gym. The great benefit of this type of equipment is how compact and light it is, making it perfect for travel.

Some exercises that you can do using an exercise band include bicep curls, upright rows and cord rows. See appendix D for full descriptions of these exercises.

Local travel

Not all travel is associated with holidays. Many businesspeople travel a number of times per week for work and they face the same challenges with staying active while away from home. The key is to incorporate some kind of formal exercise, whether it's at your hotel or a local gym, or use the hotel room workout previously discussed.

If you are just doing a day trip somewhere, factor in some sort of activity during the day. Not only will this help your weight loss, it will benefit your work performance because exercise improves your cognitive ability.

If you will be flying, apart from controlling your diet when you're on the plane, there is little you can do when you are up in the air to help you lose weight. Let's get real here, there's no way you can burn enough energy on board to make a dent into your fat deposits. If you did, the cabin crew would probably tackle and restrain you. When you are flying movement is more about maintaining good health. Get up and move enough to ensure good blood flow, especially to reduce the risk of deep vein thrombosis (DVT) during long flights. Simple leg exercises can be done while standing (often near the toilets where there is usually a little bit of room), such as calf raises or squats, or when sitting, such as foot pumps, knee lifts, heel taps and side taps. Also, wearing compression socks has been shown to reduce swelling and incidence of DVT in long-haul flights of seven to 11 hours.

Get a life

Terry was the CEO of a large company. He worked in Sydney but lived at his home in Brisbane on the weekends. Terry had become incredibly sedentary because of all the travel and long hours at work. As a result, he had put on a lot of weight and his health was suffering. When we designed his program we asked him what the key drivers were for his program. He said that he likes to have a challenge, and because he works so much he found his evenings quite boring and hadn't really established a social network in Sydney. We mapped out his program so that all of his exercise was group based and each type of exercise incorporated an event that he would be training for. For example, he joined a swim squad that met twice weekly and he signed up to do an ocean swim race. He also joined a running club and entered Sydney's huge sporting event, City to Surf. This way his program solved his two biggest needs: he was being social and he was being challenged by training for a competitive event.

Car travel

We work with a number of sales representatives who spend a huge amount of time in their cars. In terms of fat loss, this is a disaster, because most of their day is spent burning a tiny amount of energy. Doing exercise may seem impossible, but standing up during breaks and getting the blood moving is probably the most beneficial thing you can do. When you stop the car for a toilet break or to get petrol, walking around briskly will help get the blood moving. When you are in the car you can do seated exercises, such as foot pumps, knee lifts, side taps, heel taps and bicep curls. And don't forget to stretch as this reduces soreness and stiffness from remaining in prolonged positions, which makes us too sore to exercise when we get where we are going!

Keep in mind that these strategies won't help you drop lots of body fat. You must do some type of formal exercise to make up for being so sedentary and also be very mindful of your diet.

Translating tucker

In Australia, we have a few food and drink terms, like tucker, grub and tea, that can confuse even the English-speaking traveller. When we travel to a country that doesn't speak English, it is important to realise that you may not be able to find someone to translate a menu for you.

There are a couple of things you can do to ensure that you order something healthy. The old-fashioned translation dictionary has been replaced by iPhone, iPad and internet applications such as Jibbigo, which translates what you say into the local language just by talking into the microphone—like having your own personal translator. Obviously it is imperfect, but it's a good option when compared with your alternatives.

With or without a translating tool, it is a good idea to research which foods are common in the country you are visiting. Have these written in the local language, as well as pictures (more for your benefit), so you can show them to restaurant staff and limit the surprises when you get your meal.

Again, with social media, the world is becoming truly flat, so asking for help or shared experiences will allow you to prepare better for your trip abroad.

Takeaway tips

- Be aware that travelling will bring up emotional connections to holidays, and holiday eating from childhood.
- Travelling is a particularly vulnerable time for reactive eating.
- Be as prepared as you can by identifying times you will be tempted by food.
- Pre-order healthier airline options.
- Plan your eating schedule for your trip based on your schedule, duration of the trip, time zone and food availability.
- Use social media and the internet to help you find suitable locations to eat.
- Pack healthy food for your trip if appropriate.
- Pack exercise equipment and your exercise program.

Chapter 24

FIT FAMILIES

Let's revisit your priorities in life (as discussed at the begining of the book in the introduction).

You have work — check.
You are completing study or professional development — check.
You have a partner — check.
You have your family — check.
You have children — check.
You are a member of a club or service — check.
You play sports or organised exercise — check.
You have a range of activities that your children are involved in — check.
You have your faith — check.
You have hobbies — check.
You have a social life — check.
You have a virtual presence — check.

Your list of priorities could be endless, oh, and we forgot physical health. We're all still waiting for the additional 30 per cent of leisure time that Bill Gates predicted technological advances over the last two decades would provide us. Life is busier than ever before, and life is faster than ever before.

Can we have it all?

Have you ever decided to make a change in your life and then failed because *life* got in the way? When we make plans we make them with an optimistic and idealistic view rather than a realistic and optimal view. We want to have it all, and sometimes we can. At other times, priorities like our physical health simply can't override other areas of our lives. For example, when we become parents, babies can't wait for us to get home from the gym — and for that matter, neither can teenagers!

Sometimes you won't be able to be perfect. To be good enough the trick is to be as good as you can when you can, and cut yourself some slack at other times. Stressing or worrying about something that you can't change right now won't help your health. It will use up your emotional energy, which will then exhaust any resources you might have for when you do have some time to devote to your physical health. In our clinics we are amazed by the amount of time our clients devote to trying to control the uncontrollable but then don't seem concerned about making changes to the parts of their lives that are within their control.

There are a lot of busy people who have lost weight successfully. There are also a lot of super-healthy people who are CEOs of large organisations, and have children and a life.

One such *healthy* CEO is Gail Kelly. She is the CEO of Westpac and rated the eighth most powerful woman in the world by *Forbes* magazine. Now, Gail's story gets a little more interesting when you understand that she has four children. And three of those children are triplets. There are not many high-powered CEOs who could make this claim. With all of this going on, how did she rise to the top? Gail was quoted in *The Age* newspaper as saying that one key to her success was that she didn't waste time doing things to the nth degree. Having the judgement to know what is important and what isn't is what really matters to her.

The birth of kids' food

Something changed in the 1980s and 1990s. We started to see the separation of 'food' into 'kids' food' and 'adults' food'. Previously, much of the household's food was prepared at home. Cakes were baked from scratch, meals were simple and similar from day to day, and packaged snack food was almost non-existent.

It's true that life was different then and the world has significantly changed, but *really*, kids' food does not need to be different from adults' food. It's not sensible and encourages children to eat sodium- and sugar-laden snacks all day, and tempts parents to treat themselves too. We have clients who complain that their weight loss failure is due to the amount of kids' snacks filling their pantries, but realistically it's the shopping purchases in the first place that are the problem. And as we state throughout this book, it is always best to eat treats *away* from the home.

The main thing you need to remember is that there is no such thing as kids' food or adults' food. Once children are able to eat everything, they should be eating similar food to you, just in appropriate portions for their age.

Research has shown that kids eat what they like and like what they know. As we discussed in chapter 3, this is how taste preferences are developed. The Queensland University of Technology is currently studying how early child-feeding practices affect childhood obesity over time. This large, long-term study, led by Professor Lynne Daniels, is in its early stages but it's already showing promising results. At a University of Sydney lecture, Professor Daniels said, 'We need to ensure the foundations of our children's eating behaviours are set appropriately'. Food is not a toy. The majority of children know when they are full and eat to this stage if they are taught to do this.

However, to encourage children to eat more, many parents use coercion or games like flying aeroplanes, or they change the food they are feeding their child after only a few introductions because they feel that their child doesn't like the food. But the child is just not used to it yet — they are not *familiar* with it — but we know they like food they are familiar with.

Even though a sip of soft drink or a tiny spoon of sweet dessert will not directly negatively affect a child's nutritional status or weight, it may have a negative affect on their taste preferences, and the more these mini introductions occur, the more likely the baby will prefer these types of foods when they become toddlers, children, adolescents and, eventually, adults.

It is now difficult to stroll down a supermarket aisle without seeing packaging that is designed to entice children. Cartoon characters, animals and bright colours light up the aisles as though the foods are a form of decoration rather than a source of nourishment.

When today's grandparents — baby boomers — were growing up, treats like lollies, ice-cream and soft drink were offered on special occasions, such as a birthday, for everybody to share. Now kids' lunchboxes often include a treat food — every day. Kids have treat food after school, and they enjoy dessert after their meal. Three treat foods a day! This is obviously a major problem for childhood obesity, but it's also a problem for those parents who are busy and tired and want a convenient snack for themselves to pick up one of these treat foods, simply because they are exposed to them so often.

All the extra foods that we feed our kids — treat foods or otherwise — are only setting them up for health and dietary problems later in life. We tell ourselves that we are doing the best thing for them and that they will grow out of these preferences. Let us warn you — they don't. We have friends in their 30s that still don't eat vegetables, who don't eat certain meats, who never eat fruit or salads or only eat foods coated in pastry. Where do you think they learnt this from? They are not unique humans — they are just like everyone else, given special treatment by their parents who, with the best intentions, just wanted them to eat something. In our culture, food is love. In reality, food is not love.

As we have discussed throughout this book, eating treats away from home is a great way to ensure that there is no temptation to eat these foods any more frequently than as an occasional food item. Research has found that the more convenient snack and treat food is, the more you will eat it, even if you think you are eating carefully and being restrictive.

Developing healthy relationships with food is of vital importance for children. We find that many of our clients are very proactive towards their children's health but neglectful of their own health. Sometimes it may help to regard yourself as an extra child — packing lunches, serving appropriate meals and ensuring everything is balanced — just as you would for your children. If you had a child who had the kind of life you do, combined with all of your extracurricular activities, how would you plan for it? How would you make it work? I know you can make it work for your children. If you can make it work for them, you can make it work for you, too.

Family time today

The Australian Institute of Family Studies (AIFS) showed that the average father with children under five years spends around 16 hours a week with his kids, compared with 44 hours of work per week. In contrast, the average mother with children under five years spends 38 hours a week with their children and 12 hours at work. This comparison would not surprise anyone. However, it gets interesting when the child is aged over five years. After five years of age the father spends the same time at work, but his level of interaction with his children drops from 16 hours to eight hours during the week. Obviously, the children going to school and developing friendships of their own contribute to this. However, the net result is the same—parents are spending less time with their children.

As we have discussed throughout this book, our children are a major priority and it's important that the time you have available with your children is spent as quality time. Fit family strategies are a perfect way to integrate your weight loss goals with your life, without missing out on family interaction. It is the perfect productive exercise.

Exercise is a great way for a parent and child to engage and improve family bonding. In addition, this is not just a relationship issue. You know childhood obesity is a problem, and overweight kids tend to become overweight teenagers and then overweight adults.

Many factors have changed our children's level of activity. The rise of technology, increased scholastic expectations, the increased focus on child safety, parents' longer working hours, the reduction in land size, the separation from our neighbours... the list is endless.

Adam recently spoke at a conference in Fiji where small business owners came together to learn how to improve their businesses and their lives. What struck him the most was the amazing resort the conference was held in. He felt like he was in paradise. There were so many opportunities to get outdoors and be active—gorgeous beaches, beautiful pools, rock climbing, mini golf, tennis, archery, soccer and bike riding. It was paradise, with perfect weather thrown in to boot. Before his session, Adam asked one of the business owners if she was enjoying herself. She paused and said, 'We're having a bit of trouble with our son. He's refusing to leave the room and wants to go home'. Adam asked why. 'Well, there's no Foxtel here and he misses his Xbox', she replied. Adam was stunned, this kid was in paradise and all he wanted to do was stay indoors and play video games! Think of all the opportunities he was missing out on with his family to play and have fun. Being active would have been just a byproduct.

Getting the family on board

Keep in mind that when encouraging your family to get fit together, the aim isn't to force children to do anything they don't want to do. In order for them stick at being active they must enjoy the activity or the friendship group that they participate with. Find out what they like to do and see if your family time can include these activities, or at least try them out for a while. You might be surprised — what is fun for your kids, will be fun for you too. Whether it is rollerblading, backyard cricket or soccer in the park, get on board and get involved.

And remember, when you talk to children about activity and exercise use the words 'fun and play' instead.

Keep the experience positive

Parents can fall into the trap of being competitive with their kids. Egos get in the way and they have to beat their kids at the activity, or more commonly, the parents want their child to beat the other kids. Obviously this is not the way to go. Don't push your kids too hard or criticise them too much, especially when they have a coach who may already be helping them improve their sport. Kids will simply lose interest and not want to do it anymore — just like a disengaged employee. Whenever possible encourage them and point out the ways in which they are improving. Focus on their strengths.

The emotion you want them to feel is joy and excitement. Be playful with them and make the games fun. The ability to play and experience joy is a really important trait in adulthood. As we have discussed, being happy is as important as being physically healthy in terms of your longevity. However, if your kids are not naturally enthusiastic or optimistic about physical activity, you will need to encourage them. The easiest way to do this is to be a good role model. Simply exhibit enthusiasm towards being active and healthy. Children model their parents behaviour, and emotions are contagious. If you are excited and enthusiastic about going out to exercise, they will be too.

On the bandwagon

Use sporting events to spark your children's interest. When the Olympics is on, get your kids to pick their favourite athletes and let them try each of the different sports that interest them. Do this for big sporting events as well. For example, when the soccer World Cup is on, feed off this excitement and get them to experience the game for themselves. Help them to get to know the players, understand the rules and start playing with a team.

Creating a competition or making a star chart that gives the children points when they play a sporting game is one strategy. While the Olympics or another sporting event is on, like the Australian Open tennis tournament or Australian rules football or any other sports that the family is interested in watching, they can try to play as much as their favourite player or winning team. Watch a game, play a game, watch a game, play a game.

Learning and movement

Help your children to be physically active while they learn new things. Walk around with them at the zoo. Take them to a museum. Even get them to explore the local park by learning about all the bugs and animals around.

Get Santa involved

At Christmas time buy the children gifts that involve activity. Toys and games such as cricket sets, balls, bikes, scooters, skates, frisbees, hula hoops and skipping ropes not only help kids get active, they also entertain them for hours.

Entertaining the whole family

You can also keep your children's minds active while they are exercising by getting them to observe things. Try the following ideas:

- count how many steps it takes your child to go from one telegraph pole to another
- look for who sees a red car first
- count how many dogs/cats/birds you see.

Feel free to introduce some friendly competition into the family by giving everyone a pedometer and competing to see who can reach the most number of steps each day.

Takeaway tips

- There are many busy people who have stood in your shoes and still lost weight.
- You can fit in both your health and your family.
- The *best* gift you can give your children is *your* health. (I bet some of you are wishing your parents spent more time on their health when they were your age.)
- Be a positive role model. Children do what they see.
- When it comes to food or hobbies, children like what they know.
- Don't blame your kids for wrecking your diet.
- There is no such thing as kids' food.
- Continue to only have treats away from the house.
- Make family time fun by including more outdoor activities.
- Create games that include activity.
- When your children play sport, try to exercise as well.
- Create a positive family environment around exercise.

Endnote

When you start something new, it is rare that you start out being perfect at it. The same thing happens when you commit to eating well and exercising on a regular basis. We wrote *The Good Enough Diet* because we know how much pressure society puts on us to be perfect and how seriously it affects us.

In today's world we are led to believe that good is not good enough anymore. Everything has to be better, bigger, quicker, stronger and cheaper.

This is not true when it comes to weight loss. There is no benefit in setting yourself up for failure or compromising what is most important to you in your effort to have a perfect diet and exercise regimen. You will achieve great success in knowing when enough is enough, when doing what you need to do, but not more. There is success in being healthy, but not fanatical. And there is true life success in losing weight without losing your lifestyle.

We are led to believe that it's impossible to maintain our health and fitness while we build a social life or career, while we look after our children and most definitely when we travel. This is not true. You can have it all. You can lose weight, and maintain it, without losing your lifestyle.

In this book you have learned valuable lessons to help you achieve real weight loss. You now have the tools to understand what your personal priorities are and how to balance them with the essential ingredients for weight loss. And you now know what to do to make your weight loss efforts easier and ultimately more sustainable.

Yes, you do need to eat vegetables. Yes, you should exercise, but do it the right way. Yes, you might be hungry, but that's okay. Yes, you have to be proactive and plan for your success. And no, you shouldn't believe everything you hear. There will always be outrageous weight loss stories and claims, but you now know how to determine what is real and what is simply untrue.

We wish you good luck on your weight loss journey. For more meal and exercise ideas and a recommended reading list we invite you to check out our website <www.goodenoughdiet.com>.

Appendix A: Non-starchy vegetables and fruits and free flavourings

Vegetables and fruits

Throughout this book we have discussed the benefits of non-starchy vegetables and fruits. The following vegetables and fruits are low in both kilojoules and starch (carbohydrates):

- alfalfa
- asparagus
- baby spinach
- bean sprouts
- beetroot
- broccoli
- brussels sprouts
- cabbage
- capsicum
- carrots
- cauliflower
- celery
- choko
- cucumber
- eggplant
- garlic
- ginger
- green beans

- lettuce
- mushrooms
- onions
- passionfruit (limit to one per day)
- radishes
- rhubarb
- rocket
- snow peas
- spinach
- squash
- strawberries (limit to six per day)
- tomatoes
- zucchini.

Flavourings

The following list of flavourings can enhance a variety of meals:

- fish sauce
- garlic
- ginger
- herbs (for example, basil, coriander and oregano)
- liquid stock
- soy sauce
- spices (for example, chilli, cumin and tumeric)
- stock cubes
- sugar-free, oil-free salad dressings/low kilojoule salad dressing
- tomato paste
- tomato sauce
- vinegar
- worcestershire sauce.

Appendix B: Drinks and their kilojoule content

The following tables indicate the kilojoule content for a full range of flavoured drinks, from soft drinks and cordials to varieties of milk, as well as coffee drinks, alcoholic drinks and juices.

Table 1: kilojoules in flavoured drinks and milk varieties

Flavoured drinks and milk varieties	Kilojoules
Soft drink can (375 ml)	675
Soft drink bottle (600 ml)	1100
Cordial small glass (250 ml)	310
Cordial medium glass (400 ml)	480
Cordial large glass (600 ml)	750
Flavoured mineral water can (375 ml)	500
Flavoured mineral water bottle (600 ml)	800
Diet soft drink can (375 ml)	8

Table 1 (*cont'd*): kilojoules in flavoured drinks and milk varieties

Flavoured drinks and milk varieties	Kilojoules
Diet soft drink bottle (600 ml)	12
Energy drink small can (330 ml)	650
Energy drink bottle (500 ml)	975
Milk whole (250 ml)	643
Milk whole (500 ml)	1286
Milk low-fat (250 ml)	520
Milk low-fat (500 ml)	1040
Milk skim (250 ml)	365
Milk skim (500 ml)	730
Milk shake (600 ml)	1485
Thick shake (600 ml)	3300

Table 2: kilojoules in coffee drinks

Coffee drinks	Kilojoules
Latte small	561
Latte medium	739
Latte large	918
Latte skim small	318
Latte skim medium	424
Latte skim large	529
Cappuccino small	484
Cappuccino medium	623
Cappuccino large	725
Cappuccino skim small	275
Cappuccino skim medium	358

Appendix B: Drinks and their kilojoule content

Coffee drinks	Kilojoules
Cappuccino skim large	421
Mocha small	738
Mocha medium	977
Mocha large	1300
Mocha skim small	514
Mocha skim medium	684
Mocha skim large	936
Flat white small	574
Flat white medium	753
Flat white large	932
Flat white skim small	326
Flat white skim medium	431
Flat white skim large	536
Soy latte small	341
Soy latte medium	453
Soy latte large	565
Espresso	4
Short black	24
Long black	24
Long black (dash of milk)	76
Instant coffee (black)	30
Instant coffee (dash of milk)	60
Tea (black, green, herbal)	18

Table 3: kilojoules in alcoholic drinks

Alcoholic drinks	Kilojoules
Beer regular can	570
Beer regular bottle	570
Beer regular schooner	684
Beer mid-strength can	375
Beer mid-strength bottle	375
Beer mid-strength schooner	450
Beer light can	386
Beer light bottle	386
Beer light schooner	464
Beer low-carb can	450
Beer low-carb bottle	450
Beer low-carb schooner	540
Wine standard drink (100 ml)	285
Wine glass (200 ml)	570
Wine bottle (700 ml)	1995
Dark spirit and soft drink	500
Dark spirit and soda water	390
White spirit and soft drink	500
White spirit and juice	719
White spirit and soda water	390
Traditional cocktail	740
Fruity cocktail	630
Creamy cocktail	2092
Pre-mixed bottle	920
Pre-mixed can	938
Pre-mixed large can	1058

Table 4: kilojoules in juices and smoothies

Juices and smoothies	Kilojoules
Orange juice small glass (200 ml)	300
Orange juice bottle (500 ml)	750
Apple juice small glass (200 ml)	350
Apple juice bottle (500 ml)	890
Mixed juice small glass (200 ml)	375
Mixed juice bottle (500 ml)	935
Tomato juice small glass (200 ml)	180
Tomato juice large glass (500 ml)	450
Mixed vegetable juice (200 ml)	280
Mixed vegetable juice (500 ml)	600
Juice bar smoothie (no dairy) small	385
Juice bar smoothie (no dairy) medium	495
Juice bar smoothie (no dairy) large	715
Juice bar smoothie (dairy) small	925
Juice bar smoothie (dairy) medium	1300
Juice bar smoothie (dairy) large	1800

Appendix C: Example meal plans

Although we don't want to give you prescriptive meal plans, we know how much easier it is when trying to change habits to have some examples to work with. To assist you we have provided some example meal plans. You don't need to follow them perfectly, but they do include the principles we have discussed throughout this book.

When following our recipes, be experimental and try not to stick to them 100 per cent, as you can always reduce the added kilojoules and increase both the fibre and non-starchy vegetable content to suit your needs.

Example breakfasts

Breakfast is the most important meal of the day and it is important to eat something within three hours of waking. For busy people, we know how hard it is to change breakfast options daily, so we have provided four weekday and weekend choices, along with serving tips and recipes where necessary. If you already eat a healthy breakfast, you are more than welcome to stick to it. The best breakfasts include some form of

The Good Enough Diet

protein (dairy, eggs, nuts, lean meat), some non-starchy vegetables and some carbohydrate (bread, cereal, muffins). A small portion is required to lose weight. You can swap the following breakfasts options around to suit you. Table 1 provides some tasty breakfast options.

Table 1: breakfast options

Monday to Friday breakfast	Weekend breakfast	Serving tips and recipes
Bircher muesli.	Poached or boiled eggs on toast (or soldiers).	To make bircher muesli, mix 2 cups oats, ¾ cup dried fruit and 1 cup nuts/seeds (crushed). Use ½ cup of dry mix per person and add half a green apple per person and ¼ cup of berries (can be frozen). Soak ingredients overnight in ¼ cup skim milk per person. In the morning, serve with low-fat yoghurt.
Omelette made in omelette maker with added vegetables.	English muffins with ham, low-fat cottage cheese and tomato (and any other veggies you like).	See the omelette made with lots of vegetables recipe in the 'Example dinners' section.
Baked beans and ratatouille on toast.	Savoury mince on toast.	See savoury mince recipe in 'Example dinners' section. Can also serve as breakfast options in jaffles.
Avocado and tomato on toast.	Omelette with lots of vegetables.	Always use wholegrain bread for toast.

Example adult lunches

Your adult lunchbox should always include:

- *vegetables* or salad for essential nutrients and to help you feel full
- *protein* for growth, repair and recovery
- a small amount of *carbohydrate* foods for energy and bowel health.

Appendix C: Example meal plans

For optimal nutrition we have included ways you can incorporate these major food components in your lunch meals:

- *Vegetables or salad.* Can be cooked or served raw in mixed meals, such as stir fries, stews, soups or salads, or as bite-size snacks. If you are trying to lose weight, you should include more of these in your meals.

- *Protein.* Can include animal proteins (lean meat, chicken, fish, eggs, milk, cheese or yoghurt) or plant proteins (tofu, nuts, lentils, kidney beans or other legumes). Men will need more proteins in their meals.

- *Carbohydrate foods.* Includes wholegrain bread, wraps, pasta, cereal, noodles, rice, fruit, potato, sweet potato or couscous. If you are working outdoors, you will need more of these in your meals. If you are not very active (yet), you don't need to eat as much of these foods.

Table 2 provides four lunch examples each for those who work in an office and those who are more physically active throughout the day.

Table 2: sample lunches

Type of work	Example lunch 1	Example lunch 2	Example lunch 3	Example lunch 4
Office (less active)	• Tuna salad • Yoghurt • Grapes	• Lean beef and salad wrap • Apple • Nuts	• Prawns and salad • Mandarin • Yoghurt	• Chicken and vegetable stir-fry with noodles • Banana
Physical (more active)	• Pasta with meat sauce • Side salad • Muesli slice • Fruit (1 to 2 pieces)	• Ham and salad roll • Fruit (1 to 2 pieces) • Wholemeal crackers with low-fat cheese	• Tuna (medium tin) • Wholemeal crackers • Fruit (1 to 2 pieces) • Low-fat yoghurt • Veggie sticks	• Chicken and salad wrap • Fruit (1 to 2 pieces) • Low-fat muffin

If you are a lunch-skipping offender, make sure you eat at least something in the middle of the day to ensure you don't get through the entire day without eating. Skipping meals is not good for your hormones, metabolism, energy and overall health.

School lunchboxes

A recent survey found that less than 10 per cent of children's school lunchboxes meet the recommendations for a healthy lunchbox. Parents often overestimate how many treats their children should have and pack too many, often replacing an option from one of the vital food groups. Kids can also help make their lunches when they know how simple the foods are to prepare. Encourage your kids to eat at both meal breaks rather than eating everything in their lunchbox during one of the breaks, and ensure that high fibre options, including some vegetables, are provided at both breaks. This is important for kids of all shapes and sizes. Table 3 provides some ideas for lunchboxes.

Table 3: options for school lunchboxes

Dairy	Meat or alternative	Breads and cereals	Fruit	Vegetables
• 200 ml milk popper • 100 g to 200 g tub of yoghurt • 20 g to 40 g cheese	• Chicken • Tinned fish • Lean ham • Lean meat • Nuts • Egg • Small tin of baked beans	• Wholemeal bread • Rice or corn cakes • Lavash or tortillas • Rice • Pasta • Potato • Noodles • Wholemeal crackers • Air-popped popcorn • Dry high fibre cereal muesli slice • Wholemeal pancakes • Low-fat muffins	• Fresh fruit • Tinned fruit • Dried fruit • 100% fruit juice popper (not the best choice)	• Salad • Veggie sticks • Carrot • Celery • Cherry tomatoes • Cucumber • Broccoli • Celery • Vegetables in mixed meals, such as stir-fries

Using the options in table 3 as a guide, a children's healthy school lunchbox should contain:

- one to two dairy choices
- one meat or alternative food
- two to three breads and cereals
- one to two fruits
- one vegetable
- a maximum of one packaged food (optional).

Example school lunchboxes

Table 4 provides healthy and nutritious options for four school lunchboxes that will tempt even the fussiest of eaters.

Table 4: sample school lunchboxes

Example lunchbox 1	Example lunchbox 2	Example lunchbox 3	Example lunchbox 4
• Cheese and salad sandwich • Small packet of nuts • Grapes • Apple • Homemade muesli slice	• Pasta and meat sauce • Yoghurt • Banana • Mandarin • Wholemeal pancakes	• Ham and salad wrap • Low-fat milk popper • Fruit salad container • Dried apricots • Low-fat muffin	• Small tin of tuna • Ryvita or Vita-Weat crackers • Celery and carrot sticks • Mandarin • Grapes • Tub of yoghurt • Air-popped popcorn

Example dinners

The meals shown in table 5 (overleaf) are easy healthy dinner options. You don't need to be a *MasterChef* contestant to cook them, and all can be made well within half an hour.

Table 5: options for dinner

Super-quick meals	Chicken meals	Meat meals	Seafood meals	Multicultural meals
Tuna and vegetable pasta • Cook pasta (1 cup cooked per person), stir through tuna (two small tins per person) and frozen vegetables (1½ cups per person). Heat in pot on stove, or in bowls in microwave.	Chicken and noodle stir-fry • Stir-fry half a chicken breast per person, with lots of vegetables, garlic, soy sauce and oyster sauce. Add in a small amount of Hokkein noodles per person.	Kangaroo, vegetables and mashed potatoes • You can now buy kangaroo meat, including sausages, at most supermarkets. It is low-fat, but needs only a little oil to cook in pan, bake or barbecue. Use only skim milk to mash potatoes and serve a variety of other vegetables.	Fish and home-baked chips • Lightly coat fish with flour and barbecue or cook in a small amount of oil in pan. Cut up sweet potato, potato and beetroot and bake as chips. Serve with half a plate of salad.	Burritos with lots of salad • Using lean mince, mix in grated carrot and zucchini, and diced onion. Heat with burrito seasoning (bought or homemade) and red kidney beans until meat is browned. Serve in wholemeal tortillas, with avocado, tomato, lettuce, parsley, capsicum and cucumber.
Homemade pizzas • Use wholemeal pita bread, diced tomatoes or tomato paste, lots of non-starchy vegetable toppings and a small amount of low-fat cheese.	Spicy fruity chicken and salad • Cut chicken breasts in half lengthways to reduce thickness. Put on tray, cover with fruit chutney and bake in oven. Serve with salad or vegetables.	Tasty T-bones and vegetables • Use lean beef or veal T-bones and cover with very small amount of French onion soup mix. Add sliced onion. Bake in oven. Serve with lots of vegetables.	Salmon with Asian greens • Salmon is great cooked on the barbecue. While it's cooking, stir-fry Asian greens, including a variety of Chinese cabbage, beans and zucchini, in a small amount of sesame oil and soy sauce.	Spaghetti bolognaise • Using 300 g lean mince, add ¼ cup of dry red lentils with grated carrot and zucchini. Brown with onion and add a small amount of red wine. Add tinned tomatoes, herbs, tomato paste and beef stock. Serve with wholemeal pasta and a green salad.

Appendix C: Example meal plans

Super-quick meals	Chicken meals	Meat meals	Seafood meals	Multicultural meals
Savoury mince on toast • Cook 250g lean mince with 3 cups of vegetables (can be frozen), 1 dessertspoon of gravy powder, herbs and water.	Baked chicken with baked vegetables and greens • Rub chicken with a mixture of Chinese five spice powder, garlic, ginger, wholegrain mustard and water. Place on oven tray and bake. Add vegetables to tray. Serve with steamed green vegetables.	Steak and salad • Choose a lean beef, lamb or pork steak. You can bake it or cook with a small amount of oil in a pan, or barbecue. Serve with a salad.	Whole baby fish • Choose a small baby fish (e.g. flounder, baby barramundi and baby trout). Season with shallots, fresh lemon, dill, chilli and white wine. Wrap in a foil pouch and bake in a 200 degree Celsius oven for 20 to 25 minutes. Serve with a salad.	Thai green chicken and vegetable curry with brown rice • Dice chicken. Cook with onion, garlic, ginger and kaffir lime leaves until chicken is browned. Add green curry paste and cook for two minutes. Add extra vegetables (broccoli, beans, cauliflower, carrots, capsicum, celery) and coconut-flavoured skim evaporated milk. Serve with basmati rice.
Omelette with lots of vegetables • Mix two eggs per person with a dash of milk. Add in vegetables such as mushrooms, capsicum, spinach, onion, corn and tomatoes.	Chicken, pumpkin and pesto pasta • Steam or microwave 200 g pumpkin in cubes, then mash with water. Brown chicken pieces with garlic, onion and any other vegetables. Mix pumpkin and pesto with chicken and stir through pasta. Serve with a green salad.	Roast lamb with greens and roast vegetables • Choose lean cuts of meat. Season with rosemary mixed with lemon juice and garlic.	Fish and vegetable green curry • Cook 2 tablespoons of green curry paste in a pan. Dice fish, brown in pan with onion and garlic. Add vegetables, along with a tin of evaporated skim milk with a dash of coconut essence. Serve with half a cup of cooked brown rice per person.	Homemade sushi rolls • Homemade sushi (or rice paper rolls) are great fun for kids to make with you. You can buy sushi kits, which provide great ideas for recipes. To make, use sushi or brown rice, rice vinegar, with lots of vegetables and seafood.

Appendix D:
The hotel room workout

That's right, if all else fails — the weather is dreadful and there is no gym — you can use the walls and items in your hotel room. How many repetitions of each exercise you will do will depend on your fitness level. Some people can do 50 push-ups while others can only do five. Aim to do as many as you can for each exercise, but a general guideline is do 15 to 20 repetitions for each exercise and repeat each exercise twice. For bonus videos of these exercises, check out our website <www.goodenoughdiet.com>.

Wall press against a wall or push-ups on the floor

This exercise is great for your upper body. Begin by standing and facing a wall with your feet about 80 centimetres (more if you are taller) from the wall. Place your hands on the wall, shoulder-width apart. Gently lean in towards the wall by bending your elbows, keeping your body straight. Press away from the wall back to your start position and repeat.

Note: ensure that your shoulders remain back and down, keeping your neck relaxed (don't let your shoulders rise up towards your ears). To increase the intensity, perform this exercise against a table (your body will now be at a roughly 45-degree angle).

If the wall press is too easy, you can intensify the movement by doing push-ups on the floor instead. For an intermediate version, do them with your knees on the floor, like the wall press, with your body remaining straight during the movement. For an advanced version, only your toes and hands should be in contact with the floor, and again, with your body remaining straight.

Squats or sit to stand over a chair

Select a chair (bear in mind that the higher the chair the easier the exercise will be). Start by sitting on the chair with your feet flat on the floor. Stand up fully and then sit back down again, pushing your backside right back into the seat of the chair. Return to your standing position and repeat with little or no rest between movements. *Note:* you can hold hand weights during this exercise to make it a little harder. Ensure that your backside sticks out behind you and your knees remain directly above your ankles, so there is no pressure on your knee joints.

For a more intense version of this exercise, perform this same movement but without the chair behind you. From a standing position, with your feet shoulder-width apart, bend your hips and knees simultaneously to lower your backside towards the ground. Your thighs should go no lower than parallel with the ground. Again, you can hold hand weights at your side to make the exercise harder.

Tricep dips off a chair or bed

Using a chair (or bed), sit with your hands on the edge of the chair with your feet out in front of you. Move your backside off the chair and lower it towards the ground. Once your elbows get to a 90-degree angle rise back to your starting position and repeat. As you lower your body ensure that your elbows point directly behind you, and your shoulders are controlled — they should not move forwards. *Note:* the further down you go the harder the exercise will be! To make it easier or harder, move the position of your feet. Having your feet closer to the chair makes it easier.

Lunges on the spot or across the room

Standing with your feet shoulder-width apart, take a moderate step forwards. Lower yourself by bending both knees. Ensure that your back knee goes straight down towards the floor (imagine you are proposing!) and then rise up by straightening your legs. Ensure that your front knee does not go past the line of your front toes. And as for the dips, the further down you go the harder it will be! Swap legs and repeat.

The plank

- *Easy option.* Lie on the floor with your forearms bent beneath you and your palms flat on the ground. With your knees remaining on the ground, slowly raise your hips off the ground to make a straight line with your body from your knees to your shoulders. Your head stays neutral and looks at the floor.
- *Moderate option.* Assume the same position as the easy option but rather than having your knees on the ground raise them so you are resting instead on your toes and forearms. Ensure that there is a straight line between your toes and shoulders. Your head stays neutral and looks at the floor.
- *Advanced option.* Assume the same position as the moderate option. Gently raise one leg 15 centimetres off the ground and then lower to the start position. Repeat with your other leg. Continue alternating legs until you complete the time you set yourself (start with 15 seconds!). *Note:* do not rush. You don't have to hold your leg up for a long period — just a second or two. It is more important to maintain control when alternating legs.

Exercise band

One of the easiest and best pieces of exercise equipment is an exercise band. It is basically a huge rubber band that you can do just about any exercise with. It's your own portable gym. The great benefit of this type of equipment is how compact and light it is, making it perfect for travel. Overleaf are some basic rules to consider when using the exercise band.

1. Breathe continuously throughout the movement or exercise you are performing.
2. Ensure you have a firm and secure grip on the band before you begin any movement.
3. Choose the right resistance for you — if it is too easy, tighten the band by either stepping away from the anchor, or by bringing your hands closer to the anchor.
4. Use a safe anchor. Whatever you are using as an anchor (e.g. a pole, stair banister, door handle, your foot), ensure that it is secure.

Following are some simple exercises you can complete with an exercise band.

Bicep curl

Stand with your feet shoulder-width apart, with your trunk straight and holding one end of the exercise band in your hand with the other end of the band anchored beneath your foot. Holding this position, curl your hand towards your shoulders, flexing your bicep as you do this. Return to the start position and repeat on the other side.

Upright row

Stand with your feet shoulder-width apart, with your trunk straight and holding one end of the exercise band in each hand, with the middle of the band anchored beneath your foot. Holding this position, raise your arms until your hands are level with your chest, ensuring that your elbows move straight up and slightly backwards. Ensure that you keep your shoulders in the same position throughout the exercise. Return to the start position and repeat.

Cord rows

Loop the exercise band around a pole, rail or door handle that is approximately shoulder height. While facing the anchor point, stand up straight and grasp the ends of the band in each hand. From here pull the band towards you so that you slide your arms along the side of your body and your elbows end up behind your body. When you do this exercise focus on getting your back muscles to perform the movement so that your shoulder blades squeeze together.

Appendix E:
Metric to imperial conversion chart

The Good Enough Diet was written in Australia. If you are reading this in the USA, the following conversions may help.

1 calorie	=	4.2 kilojoules
1 ounce	=	28 grams
1 pound	=	454 grams
1 kilogram	=	2.2 pounds
1 mile	=	1.6 kilometres

Kilojoules	Calories	Kilojoules	Calories
418	100	4 180	1 000
1 045	250	5 225	1 250
2 090	500	6 270	1 500
3 135	750	8 360	2 000

The Good Enough Diet

Kilograms	Pounds
50	110
60	132
70	154
80	176
90	198
100	220
110	242
120	264
130	286
140	308
150	330

Grams	Ounces
50	1.75
100	3.5
200	7.0
500	17.5

Kilometres	Miles
0.5	0.3
1	0.6
2	1.2
3	1.9
4	2.5
5	3.1

Centimetres	Feet/inches
150	4, 11.0
151	4, 11.4
152	4, 11.8
153	5, 0.2
154	5, 0.6

Centimetres	Feet/inches
155	5, 1.0
156	5, 1.4
157	5, 1.8
158	5, 2.2
159	5, 2.6
160	5, 3.0
161	5, 3.4
162	5, 3.8
163	5, 4.2
164	5, 4.6
165	5, 5.0
166	5, 5.4
167	5, 5.7
168	5, 6.1
169	5, 6.5
170	5, 6.9
171	5, 7.3
172	5, 7.7
173	5, 8.1
174	5, 8.5
175	5, 8.9
176	5, 9.3
177	5, 9.7
178	5, 10.1
179	5, 10.5
180	5, 10.9
181	5, 11.3
182	5, 11.7
183	6, 0.0
184	6, 0.4
185	6, 0.8

Index

advice
— advertising 147, 148
— amateur 146, 147
— appropriate 145-6, 147, 148, 150
— assessing 147-9, 150
— claims too good to be true 149-150
— commercial 147-8, 149
— internet 146, 147, 149
— practicality 147, 148
— professional 146
— research behind 147-8, 149, 150
aerobic (cardiovascular) exercise 80, 81
alcohol 7, 50, 53, 186-7, 192, 214
— *see also* wine
all or nothing dieting xiii-xiv, xvi, vxiii
anxiety 34, 38
Asian meals 18, 19, 176
audiobooks 61

balance approach xiii-xiv, xvi-xix
balance bar graph xviii-xix, 150
barriers to weight loss 1-2, 14
behaviour 117-21
— four levels of interpretation 117-21
— *see also* emotions
blood glucose 37, 87, 94, 152
bone density 78
boredom 12, 15-16, 23, 27, 28, 34, 35, 71, 100, 135, 137-8
bowels 43, 147, 187, 218
brain-derived neurotrophic factor (BDNF) 59-60
bread 25, 27, 28, 91, 151, 153, 155, 174, 175, 180, 186, 187, 189, 218, 219, 220, 221
breakfast 19-20, 29, 139, 161
— ideas 19-20, 154, 159, 217-218
business meetings
— exercise 75, 79, 93, 133
— food xii, 8, 9, 11, 16, 31, 47, 48-9, 58-9, 158

Caesar salad 174-5
cake 11, 40, 59
— carbohydrates 145, 153-4, 155, 156
cardiovascular exercise *see* aerobic exercise
carbohydrates 145, 153-4, 155, 156, 180-1
case studies
— children 137-8
— exercise 58-9, 60-1, 92-4, 95-6, 165, 192, 195

— food and weight loss xiii-xiv, 8-10. 16-17, 24-6, 32-3, 40-1, 47-9, 137-8. 152-3, 158-60, 172-3, 177-8,
— health myths 146
— mindset 126-7, 130-1
— travel 172-3, 189, 192, 195
chafing 110-11
chewing 140-1
children xx, 19, 125, 137-8
— exercise 59, 92-4, 203-6
— food habits 11, 18, 19, 135-6, 139, 201-2
— hunger 135-8
— kids food 200-2
— lunches for 29, 220-2
— obesity 125, 137-8
— retraining food habits 135-8
— variety 27-8
clothing, exercise 105-9, 110, 111
coffee 48, 49, 51-2, 212-13
combining food *see* food combining
comfort food 31-8
compression garments 110-11
condiments 174-5, 182
cooking methods 43, 46
cravings 37-8, 43, 154

Deep Vein Thrombosis (DVT) 195
diet drinks 52, 53, 211-12
dietary guidelines xii, 21, 26
diet foods 39, 40
diets and weight loss, xv
dining out *see* eating out
dinners, healthy 179-81, 222-3
— *see also* eating out; meals
discrimination, 123-4
dressings 175, 182
drinks 47-53
— flavoured 211-12
— kilojoule content 48, 49, 50, 51, 53, 211-15
— requirements 51-2
— sugar content 49
— weight loss 48, 52, 53
— *see also* alcohol; coffee; cordial; energy drinks; juice; milk; probiotic drinks; soft drinks; sports and energy drinks; tea; wine

eating, retraining habits 135–41, 156
eating out xviii, 3, 7, 14, 21, 26, 29, 52, 171, 172–5
— healthy 172–6
— *see also* free meal
emotional eating 31–5, 98, 157, 197
— strategies to manage 35–8
emotions 97–9, 116, 121
— motivation 99–101
— *see also* emotional eating; mindset
energy drinks 10, 212
energy slumps 94, 152–3
— sweet cravings 152–3
— *see also* snacks
excuses xi–xii, 4, 7, 66, 67, 68, 72–3
exercise and weight loss 11–12, 80–1, 57–111
— amount of 76–8
— changing habits 65–73, 101–2
— cold weather 108–9
— combining with business 59–61, 62–3, 92, 93
— combining with social life 62–3, 66, 68, 70, 100, 102
— emotions 62, 97–102
— equipment 193, 197, 227–8
— excuses 66, 67, 68, 72–3
— family 93–4, 204–6
— four principles 78–84
— friction problems 107, 108, 110–11
— fun 62, 66, 68, 69, 62–3, 66, 68, 70, 97–103
— goals 68, 102
— guidelines 76–7, 165
— hot weather 106–8
— illness, 109–10
— incidental 88–92, 132
— injuries 72, 73, 100, 109, 111, 167
— intensity 79–81, 163–7
— learning, effect on 59–60
— making time for 25, 57–9, 60–3, 79, 92–6, 102, 132
— motivation 99–101
— office 92–6
— overdoing 67, 68–9
— personality profiles 65–73
— productivity 92–6
— starting 101–2
— teams 62, 96, 100–1, 102, 132–3
— technology and 60–3
— third space, 129–34
— timing 76, 78–9, 87–96
— variety 69
— with others 62–3, 66, 68, 70
— *see also* clothing for exercise; fat burning zone; hotel room workout; interval training; resistance training; trainers and sports professionals

fad diets 3, 15, 17, 23, 24, 118, 150, 151, 177
failure, sense of xii, xviii
— *see also* self-sabotage
family, healthy 199–206
— activity 203–6
— exercise 93–4, 204–6
— kids food 200–2
— time for 203–4, 206
— *see also* children
fast food, healthy 171, 176–8
fat burning zone 163–7
fats 41, 45, 147, 153, 154, 155, 156
— benefits in weight loss 43–5
— good vs bad 43–5
— hidden 174–5
— *see also* low-fat foods
fibre 51, 174, 180, 217
flavourings, food 210
— *see also* condiments; sauces; spreads
food combining 151–5
— benefits of 151
— carbohydrates 145, 153–4, 155, 156
— carbohydrates and protein 153, 154, 156
— fat content 153, 154, 174–5
— proteins 145, 153–4, 155, 156
food diary 141
food groups 20, 26, 27, 153–4, 220
footwear for exercise 108
free meal 13, 14, 43
freezing food tips 181–2
French diet 39, 42
frozen dinners 181–2
frozen vegetables 21, 22, 180
fruits, list of suitable 209–10

guilt xix, 27, 32, 34, 41, 95, 99

habits, breaking *see* children; retraining
health halo 41–2, 91
health in a hurry 171–84
heat stress 106–7
home-delivered meals 178–9
hotel room workout 194, 225–7
hunger 153
— boredom and 15–16, 71, 137–8
— brain vs belly 36–7, 138
— causes 153
— children 135–9
— embracing 139–41
— is okay 135–42
— re-learning 138–9

Index

—warm meals 36-7
—*see also* emotional eating; reactive eating; proactive eating
hydration 51-2, 107-8, 149, 187

Indigenous health 32
in-flight meals 9, 187-8, 189, 197
—*see also* travel
intensity of exercise 163-7
interval training 79-81, 165
iPod and exercise 60-1, 103

joint problems 109, 111
juice 51, 215
junk food 7, 189, 33, 34, 189

kids *see* children
kilojoules not fats 39, 41, 42

learning and exercise 59-60
life balance *see* work–life balance
love, food as 33, 43, 138, 141, 202
low-carbohydrate diets 15
low-fat foods 39-46
    —energy slumps 152-3
    —kilojoule content 39, 40, 41, 42, 43, 152-3, 156
    —no-fat foods 42
    —recommended 42
lunch
    —adult 218-20
    —children's 29, 220-22
    —*see also* meal plans and planning: meals
lycra bike pants, benefits of 110

meal plans and planning 8, 9, 10-11, 12-13, 14, 23, 25, 27, 28
    —adult lunch 218-20
    —breakfast 217-18
    —children's lunches 220-1
    —dinners 221-3
    —sample 217-23
    —variety 25-7
    —weekly plan 179
meals 12-13, 14, 27, 157
    —healthy choices 171-84, 220-1
    —lunchbox ideas 220-2
    —number of 157-61
    —on a plate 20, 139-40
    —timing 138-9
    —travelling 172-3, 176, 178, 188-9
    —unhealthy choices 174-5
    —*see also* breakfast; dinners; in-flight meals; eating out; free meal; lunch; snacks; travel; treats

medication 77, 116
meditation and exercise 62, 63
milk 149, 211-12
mindset 34, 36, 57, 115-42
    —changing 2, 36, 124-7, 130
    —consistency 116-17
    —*see also* behaviour; emotions
mirror affirmations 128
misconceptions *see* myths
monounsaturated fats 43, 45
myths, health and weight loss 115-16, 145-67
    —*see also* advice; fat burning zone

negotiation with self 35, 38, 75-6, 138
nuts, 44, 45, 46

obesity 124-5, 137-8
oils for cooking 20, 44, 46
omega-3 fats 43, 44, 45
overeating 20, 34, 35, 136, 158-61, 189
    —strategies to avoid 35-8
    —*see also* emotional eating; hunger

pantry, fridge and freezer suggestions 180-1
pasta 18, 25, 29, 151. 155, 174, 175, 180, 181, 182, 219, 220, 221, 222, 223
personal trainers *see* trainers and sports professionals
Pilates 84
planning to lose weight 11-13
    —*see also* meal plans and planning; meals; proactive eating; travel
plates 20, 139-40, 141
polyunsaturated fats 43, 45
portion size and portion control 2, 21, 22, 36, 41, 42, 45, 138, 139, 153, 154, 156, 157, 160, 172, 173, 175, 176, 178, 179, 181, 182, 184, 189, 190, 201, 218
    —*see also* serving size and proportions
pressure, self-imposed xx
priorities xvii, xix, 4, 13, 24, 199, 200, 208
proactive eating 7-14
probiotic drinks 187
proteins 37, 43, 145, 153-4, 155, 156, 174
    —choices 180-1
    —*see also* food combining; serving size and proportions

quick fixes 148, 150, 151
    —*see also* fad diets; pills, weight loss

reactive eating 7, 10, 13, 37, 43, 197
    —low-fat foods 40-1, 43, 45
recipes 222-3
rehydration *see* hydration

resistance (weight) training 81–4, 100–1, 165, 167
retraining eating habits 136–42, 156
rice 19, 26, 28, 29, 151, 155, 156, 174, 175, 176, 180, 183, 219, 220, 223

sabotaging yourself *see* self-sabotage
salads 19, 20, 21, 22, 25, 27, 36, 152, 174–5, 177, 180, 181, 182, 186, 187, 189, 202, 210, 218, 219, 220, 221, 222, 223
sandwiches *see* bread
satiety 42–3
sauces 175, 182
segmenting your life 133
self-acceptance 124–8
self-esteem 124–8
self-loathing 123
self-sabotage xviii, 11, 35, 118, 128, 150
self-suggesting 19, 124–8
self-talk 127–8
serving size and proportions 21, 41, 173–4, 175, 176, 218, 219
— carbohydrates 155, 218, 219
— fats 174
— fibre 174
— healthy foods 41–3, 175–6
— low-fat foods 40, 41–3
— non-starchy vegetables 15, 16, 21, 22, 139, 140, 156, 172, 173–4, 175
— proteins 155, 174, 218, 219
— proteins + carbohydrates 156
— *see also* portions and portion control
shopping strategies 8, 13, 26, 29, 171, 179, 182–3, 201
situational meals and plans 8–10, 11
smoothies 215
smorgasbord syndrome 28, 29, 186
snacks 21, 136, 152–3, 186–7, 189, 201
— ideas for healthy 154–5, 160
soft drinks 49, 211
sports and energy drinks 10, 107, 147, 212
spreads 19, 44, 45, 46
sugar and dieting 15
supplements 37, 44, 147
support team 8–9, 13, 14, 17, 131, 178, 179

taste preferences 20, 22, 201
— strategies to change, 17, 18–19
— *see also* retraining eating habits
tea 51–2
technology and weight loss 1, 2, 10–1, 60–1, 103, 182–3
third space and exercise 129–34
time-saving tips 171–84
— eating out 172–5
— fast food, healthy 171, 176–8
— frozen dinners 181–2
— home-delivered meals 178–9
— online shopping 182–4
— pantry, fridge and freezer suggestions 180–1
— quick dinners 179–81, 222–3
trainers and sports professionals 67, 72–3, 105, 145
travel, weight loss and 172–3, 176, 178, 185–97
— airport food choices 185–7
— alcohol 186–7, 192
— car 195–6
— exercise 191–4, 195, 197
— healthy eating 172–3, 176, 178, 186
— hotel room workout 194, 225–7
— hydration 187
— in-flight meals 9, 187–8, 189, 197
— local 194–6
— meals 172–3, 176, 178, 192
— plans 173, 188–9
— reactive eating, 197
— sleeping times 188
— taking food along 189, 190–2, 197
— technology 191, 196, 197
— time zone management 187–8
treats 7, 43, 176, 192, 202
— healthy 42–3
— planning 12–13, 28, 38, 43

variety 17, 18, 20, 23–9
— less for weight loss 23–4, 25–8
vegetables 21, 180–1
— *see also* vegetables, non-starchy
vegetables, non-starchy 15–22, 28, 29, 37, 139, 140, 156, 172, 174, 175, 176, 180–1, 184, 189, 218
— list of 209–10
— *see also* salads; serving size and proportions
vegetarian protein 180, 219

walking and weight loss 17, 58–9, 63, 76, 79, 80, 81, 90, 93, 100, 102, 109, 135, 164, 165, 166, 167, 192, 193, 196
warm food and drink 36–7, 52
weight-loss pills 1, 15, 148, 150
willpower 69, 70, 77, 117, 118, 124
wine 48, 49, 50, 60, 115, 116, 120, 186, 187, 214, 222
work–life balance xiv, xvi–xix, 3–4, 129–33

yoga 84

www.ingramcontent.com/pod-product-compliance
Lightning Source LLC
LaVergne TN
LVHW010255260326
834688LV00044B/1301